Endorsements

Nancy Poland was fortunate to grow up with a father who was truly one of the greats of the Greatest Generation, yet she shares the misfortune of so many: loving a parent who succumbed to the elusive and inescapable effects of Lewy Body dementia. In these pages she shares her family's struggles and triumphs and illuminates the path so others can better navigate the vagaries of American dementia care.

Judy Cornish, Esq.,Founder of the Dementia & Alzheimer's Wellbeing Network® (DAWN) and the DAWN Method®, Author of *The Dementia Handbook* and *Dementia With Dignity, Living Well with Alzheimer's or Dementia Using the DAWN Method*

This compassionate and resource heavy book will be a beacon to families living with Lewy Body Dementia. Ms. Poland's insights as a daughter are invaluable. The details of the progression of the disease may be helpful for others walking this path. An important light into a rarely understood disorder.

Diane W. Carr, Masters in Public Health, Patient Navigator, retired, Be The Match / National Marrow Donor Program

"Dancing with Lewy" offers practical advice to caregivers, who have to deal with myriad of personal, medical, financial, and legal issues. Nancy clearly stated the importance of maintaining the oral hygiene of patients suffering from diseases such as Lewy Body Dementia and Parkinson's. As a dentist who has treated patients suffering from dementia and Parkinson's, I totally agree. A healthy, disease free oral cavity is an important component of optimal whole-body wellbeing. Also, Nancy Poland stresses the importance that the caregivers have to take care of themselves to be effective.

Eugene G Dvoracek DDS, a retired family practice dentist

If you want helpful resources and tips for caregivers of afflicted loved ones, "Dancing with Lewy" covers it all. While dementia creates heartache and struggle this book portrays highlights of the American Dream era with vivid pictures of the author's growing up years. Memories and reflections interspersed with poetry written by her father captured me completely. An honest and transparent journey of a loving daughter who remembers the joy, but also struggles with exhaustion, crankiness, and guilt. A must read for every caregiver out there.

Marianne Foscarini, Christian Copywriter

Nancy Poland has given us a creative, compassionate, honest and emotional work on a family journey with a father who has Lewy Body Dementia. I found this fine book stirring up all kinds of emotions as my family journeyed with my father who had Parkinson's disease. I could not put the book down and I think that would be your experience if you pick up and read this book!

Mark Hovestol (Retired Pastor and College President)

Having lost my mother to dementia within the past year, I can only say I wish Nancy Poland's book, "Dancing with Lewy", could have been published sooner. You will laugh, cry, be serenaded by her father's poetry and emerge better equipped to find joy in your journey through the dementia of a parent, patient or loved one. Her kind and compassionate story promises comfort and insights for caregivers and family members in distress.

Marnie Swedberg, Author, Leadership Mentor

dancing with LEWY

NANCY R. POLAND

dancing with LEWY

A Father-Daughter Dance
Before and After Lewy Body
Dementia Came to Live With Us

NEW YORK
LONDON • NASHVILLE • MELBOURNE • VANCOUVER

Dancing with Lewy

A Father-Daughter Dance, Before and After Lewy Body Dementia Came to Live with Us

Published in New York, New York, by Morgan James Publishing. Morgan James is a trademark of Morgan James, LLC. www.MorganJamesPublishing.com

ISBN 9781631951275 paperback
ISBN 9781631951282 eBook
Library of Congress Control Number: 2020935959

Cover Design by:
Megan Dillon
megan@creativeninjadesigns.com

Interior Design by:
Christopher Kirk
www.GFSstudio.com

Disclaimer
This is a memoir based on the author's memories of events. While all experiences relayed actually occurred, some names and identifying details have been changed to protect the privacy of individuals and businesses.

Dedication Page

For my three sisters who loved and cared for our Dad every step of the way. You have each made the world a better place, and I am blessed to have you in my life.

Table of Contents

Preface

Don't look back, friend; look ahead
You'll meet the living, not the dead.
Soldiers meet the enemy face-to-face,
They don't run a backward race.
If you can't find the enemy up ahead,
It's because you stopped fighting, and, friend, you're dead.
'Cause in this life, the enemy's there;
You may not always know just where.

So make up your mind, the hour is late,
Some battles are small, and some are great
You'll be fighting God's battle right up to the gate.
So lead on, warrior, and don't despair,
'Cause at the end of the battle we'll all be there.

All poetry is from the family's booklet,
"Memories in Verse – the Poems of Lee E. Eggerud".
The poems are original with minor grammatical corrections.

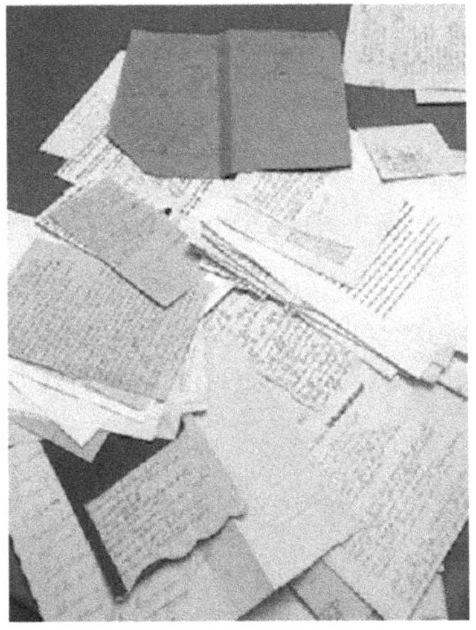

How Dad Wrote his Poetry

Acknowledgments

Many people played a part in this story.

Life-long gratitude goes to my mom and dad, who loved me unconditionally, taught me compassion, and showed me in an imperfect way the faithfulness of a perfect God.

My husband John, who has stood by me and cheered me on for over 40 years. He brought my parents to doctor appointments, picked up medications and listened to their stories. John had hot meals waiting for me at home after long nights in the nursing home with Dad. And he held me while I grieved.

I am so grateful for our sons Lee and Corey, who encourage me and remind me of the goodness of life.

A big thank you to my sisters who provided photos, clarified the timing of events, and reminded me of how to love when times were the most difficult.

A special thank you to Terri, who proofread this manuscript multiple times, and to readers Marcia and Diane, who provided content input.

My professional team: Barbra Kois, copy editor, Mariya Anderson, photo editor and Brittany Cahoy, photographer were thoughtful and supportive.

Thank you to Terry Whalin and Morgan James Publishing for believing in me.

Most of all thanks be to God for the gifts of grace, mercy and hope for a future of no more pain and suffering.

Part I –

Our Story

Chapter 1
The End

The church was hushed. He lay there still, quiet. At least now I didn't have to see his vacant eyes.

How often had I stared into twinkling bright blue eyes when he told a good story? Where was the little half smile and throaty chuckle I heard when he tried to hold back laughter at his own jokes?

I even missed his warm breath, tinged with the scent of coffee.

What was the difference between his state now and his state just days before? He had not been living, just existing for the past fourteen months. Then and now—still, quiet, vacant.

The tears wouldn't come, just an all-enveloping sadness. Sadness, regret, and anger. A hundred whys.

Why did my dad, Lee, have to suffer from this illness? Dad,

fiercely independent, a self-made businessman, kind and loving—why did this happen to his brain?

Why didn't I ask him more about his childhood when he could talk?

Why did Lewy steal our last years with Dad?

Why did I resent him telling me how to live my life?

Why did I harbor hardness in my heart about the past?

I was the last one to walk up to the coffin before they closed the lid. Seventy pairs of eyes watched me. The perfume of flowers penetrated the air.

I touched his hand; it was stiff. An odd thought came into my head: Dad wasn't supposed to have stiff hands. He was strong, even at the end his grip startled the nursing aides. His hands held his babies, measured and cut ceiling tile, carved wooden signs, and delicately repaired glass and crystal.

Now his hands were artificially folded over his heart.

We had our "final words," my father and me. I spoke and imagined he agreed. What I did not know was how those final words would forever change me.

Words I wished I could have said to him years ago.

Words that heal, and the healing continues now, years later.

I will tell you those words later.

Lewy

Lewy—I did not know his name until right before he struck his final blow. When exactly Lewy first came into our family is unknown. I do know that Lewy body dementia is a horrible, destructive disease, a destroyer of lives.

(I'm calling Lewy a "he" because it was named after a man. However, Lewy body dementia is no respecter of persons: male, female, rich, poor, whatever race or religion.)

This is a bittersweet story of my dance with Lewy body dementia ("Lewy"). This is also a father-daughter story of my dad and me, before and after Lewy came to live with us.

Stay with me and you will read the story of the young Lee, growing up in the Depression years. He became a self-made business owner, the father of four daughters. You will read how Dad and I carefully danced around each other for many years, but especially when dementia stole his mind and body.

The story, however, is not always sad.

There are moments of humor and hope.

Precious memories.

The promise of seeing Dad again in a place where there is no Lewy or tears of sorrow.

It is the story of grace.

This story is my memoir, my truth revealed to you, as well as I recall. Perhaps you will feel my raw emotions. I'll be honest with you, even when you question my decisions or motives.

I have taken a bit of literary license to make the story relevant for the times. There may be a bit of drama for emphasis. However, I am Scandinavian and from Minnesota—we are known for our natural reserve. So not too much extra drama!

I believe my father, the great storyteller, would approve of me telling our story.

What is Lewy body dementia and who made this discovery?

When Dr. Friederich H. Lewy was working in Dr. Alois Alzheimer's laboratory he made an important discovery as described in the Lewy Body Dementia Association website:

> *In the early 1900s, while researching Parkinson's disease, the scientist Friederich H. Lewy discovered abnormal protein deposits that disrupt the brain's normal functioning. These Lewy body proteins are found in an area of the brain stem where they deplete the neurotransmitter dopamine, causing Parkinsonian symptoms. In Lewy body dementia, these abnormal proteins are diffused throughout other areas of the brain, including the cerebral cortex. The brain chemical acetylcholine is depleted, causing disruption of perception, thinking and behavior. Lewy body dementia exists either in pure form, or in conjunction with other brain changes, including those typically seen in Alzheimer's disease and Parkinson's disease.*[1]

There you have a mini-scientific explanation. It falls short of the physical toll ravaging body and mind. It doesn't touch the emotional and financial impact on families.

Lewy body dementia has elements of Parkinson's disease, such as rigidity. Some Parkinson's patients experience hallucinations; however it is a more common sign of Lewy body dementia. Lewy may bring brain confusion like Alzheimer's, although there are not always the memory issues. Ultimately, Lewy delivers the immobility brought by amyotrophic lateral sclerosis (known as ALS or Lou Gehrig's disease).

Until we were well into my dad's dementia, I had heard very little about Lewy body dementia. My first exposure to the disease was when my friend Karen's husband became forgetful, angry, and stubborn. Karen was confused; Danny, her mild-mannered husband in his early sixties, had never exhibited such behavior. They went from doctor to doctor, seeking a solution.

Initially, Danny was diagnosed with Lewy body dementia, an unusual name for a disease. I learned about Lewy from Karen. My husband befriended Danny; when they went out for lunch my husband ordered and managed the payments. When Danny entered the nursing home, my husband faithfully visited him and watched him deteriorate mentally and physically. Eventually they concluded that Danny did not have Lewy body dementia; he was latently diagnosed with frontal-lobe dementia. Lewy and other dementias are sneaky and deceitful.

Danny died in his sixties and Karen became a widow. At his funeral, she played "Somewhere Over the Rainbow." I like to think of Danny, who loved to sing in the church choir and always had a smile and a handshake for everyone, happy and free on the other side.

Celebrities reportedly having Lewy body dementia include:

- The great comedian Robin Williams committed suicide, possibly related to his undiagnosed dance with Lewy. Robin suffered from depression, anxiety, and delusions. Lewy imparts those symptoms on its victims. Robin Williams' widow wrote about Lewy in "The Terrorist Inside My Husband's Brain". [2]
- One of my best teen memories is driving around listening to Casey Kasem's "Top 40." Casey Kasem's voice was silenced because of Lewy. That is another insidious trait of Lewy, silencing its victims. I cried when I heard of this diagnosis that tore his family apart.
- Ted Turner, founder of CNN, revealed he has Lewy body dementia. While on *60 Minutes*, he could not remember the name of the disease because Lewy steals the memory. Like my dad, he did not think this was that bad of a disease.

Perhaps the only good to come out of these diagnoses is that Lewy body is becoming better known. While there are no cure and few treatments for Lewy, there is hope in research.

If I am ever diagnosed with Lewy body dementia, don't tell me.

The dance is not always with your loved one; it is a dance around the disease. At times it is a slow dance; at times it is a tap dance. And sometimes when we dance, we trip over our own two feet.

Albert Einstein is believed to have said:

> *"We dance for laughter, we dance for tears, we dance for madness, we dance for fears, we dance for hopes, we dance for screams, we are the dancers, we create the dreams."*

This is our dance with Lewy.

Chapter 2

A Look Back

I was born in Brainerd fair, where the hills and trees
Sometimes, yet beckon to me-
A long time ago in the far distant past
I stored them, in my memory, by making a poem,
And filed them away to remember my home.
And the years that have passed
and the things I have dared,
Are treasures that maybe no troubadour has sung.

But poets are different—they'll find something to write
About any subject whether the morning or the night.
So if I was tilling the soil or sailing the sea,
A poem can store its memory for me.

I'm so grateful to have the heart of a poet,
Today I would like the whole world to know it.

Why was my Dad such a hard worker? What made him become an entrepreneur?

In this chapter you will meet the young man who made my dad the man he became.

Dad was part of the "Greatest Generation." Born in 1926, he grew up in Brainerd, a small town in north central Minnesota.

The Great Depression years formed him, the son of a farmer, the fourth child of nine siblings.

Family stories bind us together and give us hope for each new generation. When I was young, I did not appreciate the hardiness of my great-grandparents, who came to America, or my grandparents and my parents, who lived through the World Wars, the Great Depression, and the building of America.

I stand in awe of my ancestors, building this country from scratch. In some ways we are such wimps now. I whine if my dishwasher quits working or the internet is out for an hour!

I've captured a few stories here and will weave in others throughout the narrative. You will see how the times formed my dad and so many in his generation. Details are filled in by my aunt's writing about her younger brother, my dad, in a genealogy book and in a letter my dad wrote to his niece when his oldest brother died.

My aunt described my dad as follows: "Never have I known a child or a man with so much genuine love in his heart for his fellow man. I have never known him to be unkind, untrue, or mean-spirited toward anyone, human or animal. I trusted him implicitly during our growing up years; I trust him still. I am one year and two months his senior, but it is I who now, on occasion, look to him for advice and consolation. He has become my big brother. One to respect, one to love. I count my blessings."

My dad described country life in this poem:

Water from the well, the lamps were kerosene,
'Twas the finest life that you have ever seen.
Milk was from the cow, and eggs from the hen,
I think that things were better for us then.
Horses in the barn, cars were always old,
Houses not the finest, winters mostly cold.
School was miles down the road, snow was always deep.

These are memories in my heart that I shall always keep.
After school and work, bones and feet were aching,
Half a mile down the road, you could smell bread a'baking.
Soup cooking in the kettle, pie in the oven
Add this all together, and you've got country.

Everyone worked on the farm, whether it be in the big garden, cooking, feeding the chickens, pumping water, caring for the horses or cows, or keeping track of the younger kids. When they were old enough, they looked for work outside the farm. Dad and his older brother sold newspapers, the *Minneapolis Tribune* (the predecessor to the current *Star Tribune*).

The boys would arrive at the paper office early in the morning to pick up the papers. During the summer tourist season, they would sell the paper at intersections in town, at the bus station, and in restaurants. The papers sold for about two cents each. Sometimes the owners would take the boys swimming if they sold the supply by mid-afternoon. On hot days it was a pleasant reward.

Sometimes they stayed in town overnight, sleeping in the paper room. They would lie on a pad of papers and cover up with sheets of the news. "It does keep you warm, but sort of hard to keep covered, and not too good a mattress," Dad reported.

Another entrepreneurship endeavor involved lefse, a Norwegian concoction of potatoes, cream, and flour, rolled thin and cooked on a big grill. We smother warm lefse with sugar and cinnamon. Grandma would make a basketful of lefse, and the kids would sell it in town. No one could make lefse like Grandma. One time my dad was rolling out the lefse for Thanksgiving dinner. His mom, my grandma, snatched the rolling pin from Dad. "No, Lee, it's got to be thin—like this!"

Back in the country, the boys would also chop down wood, gather scrap metal, and trap fur-bearing animals. They sold these items in town. I see why my dad became a business owner later in life—he learned young to make his own way.

Dad admitted in the letter that they did some "bad" things at times, for example, sneaking away for an afternoon movie, such as *Flash Gordon* or the *Lone Ranger*. Or they would buy Wing cigarettes which were long and cheap. They'd sneak out behind buildings to smoke.

Grandma warned the kids *not* to pick up cigarettes thrown out of cars, as they were probably "dope" meant to get kids hooked. (Dad said they could never figure out how "they" would know who found them and became hooked.)

Childhood Disasters

When Dad's older sister was five and he was four, they found a kitchen match their dad had accidentally left on his workbench after repairing an inner tube for the Ford.

The kids hoped to find somewhere to play and settled on the barn. If they could clean out the hay, there would be lots of room! They climbed up the ladder leaning against the inner wall of the barn to get to the hayloft. Dragging hay from the middle of the loft to the corner, they figured they could get a good blaze going.

It was his sister who struck the match; the kids watched as the flames took hold and started climbing to the top of the pile. Suddenly, the prospect of what was happening hit her five-year-old "gray matter" and down they went, running at breakneck speed to get as far away as possible from the barn.

My aunt's first thought was to go into hiding, thinking she could escape her mother's discipline.

My four-year-old dad, on the other hand, ran into the house to tell. Their mother was horror stricken! She became frantic and ran toward the barn, trying to find my aunt, who was eventually found peeking under the front porch.

Cars stopped along the road to help put out the fire. A couple hundred chickens died. Fortunately, the sole cow had been tied up away from the barn. After the excitement was over, my aunt recalled her mother giving her several sound swats with the butter paddle. No swats for Dad, however. Grandma knew he was not the culprit; after all, it was he who came to report the misdeed.

My aunt described the event as "an *uffda* for sure for our mother."

(In case you are not familiar with "uffda," it is a handy Norwegian expression used when a person is baffled, dismayed, or surprised.)

I can only imagine all the near disasters that can happen with nine kids. (I spent plenty of time in the emergency room or urgent care with only two boys!) Miraculously, all nine lived to adulthood.

At one time, my dad had an almost fatal accident. His older brother syphoned gas out of the tank of the car with a hose. My dad, the younger brother, thought he would try this trick. Unfortunately, he inhaled fumes and had a horrible reaction. His parents grabbed little Lee, jumped in the car, and raced to town to the doctor's office, where they pumped his stomach.

Another time, Dad's oldest brother acquired an infection on his chin, which turned into streptococcus in his bloodstream. There were no antibiotics back then. The doctor said there was no cure other than a transfusion from someone who had recovered from such an infection. The only case they knew of was out East, and being during the Depression, they had no money. He was certain to die.

Grandma and Grandpa brought their son to church, and the pastor prayed that Jesus would heal him. They anointed him with oil, as prescribed in the Bible. The boy became very ill and threw up what looked like gobs of black blood. He was healed, and the pastor continued to recount this story sixteen years later. Yes, God does answer prayer.

Another one of the brothers was hit by a pitchfork, and two tines went right into his head. Another brother pulled it out, along with a lot of blood. Another race to the doctor!

The kids had ringworm, pneumonia, scarlet fever, and a whole variety of other illnesses. Sometimes Grandma would barely sleep for a whole week tending to ill family members. It's amazing all nine kids lived into adulthood.

Although times were tough, I must believe that these family disasters created our calm, cool dad. He seldom got riled and seemed to never be afraid. I remember him taking me to the emergency room for stitches; his composure calmed me down.

He wasn't afraid until much later, when Lewy came into our lives.

Family Fun

But back to the early days—there were also fun family times.

When not working, the family spent summers swimming and boating. Often, when their dad came home from work on a hot summer evening, the family would take picnic baskets, pile into the car, and go to the lake for supper and swimming.

In winter there was sledding, tobogganing, and skiing. Grandpa made a strong and beautifully handcrafted toboggan; it lasted from their childhood days to those years when grandchildren came to the farm for vacation.

The winter cold and long and bleak,
I think may end sometime this week.
Maybe summer then will come,
Seems my brain is frozen numb.

I sure don't care where winter goes,
Or where she hides her frozen snows.
Just help me find that dear old sun,
And let's all have some summer fun.

They hunted, learned to drive the old Ford, played baseball, and acted in plays at school. When they were older, they attended school dances and dated. Riding horses bareback—sometimes without even a halter, through the wooded areas and over the wide-open fields that lay between the farm and that of their closest neighbors—was a highlight of their youth.

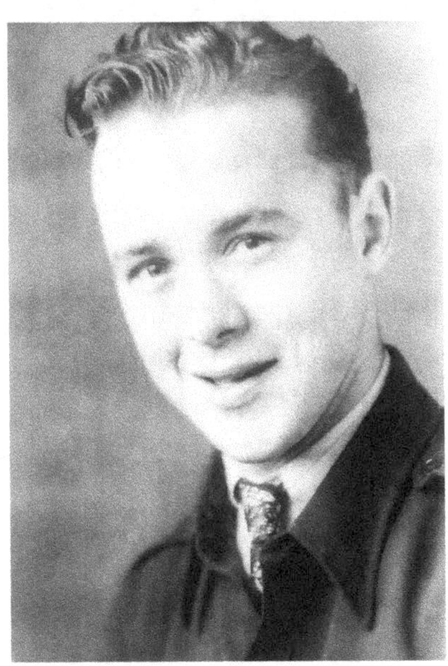

Dad in his Teens

Grandma

Dad loved to talk about his mom. She made certain the kids were at church whenever possible. The girls got to wear their dresses, and the boys pulled on their itchy wool pants. If the kids wriggled too much, "Ma" (Grandma) would pull their ears. I can just picture her surrounded by kids, keeping them all in line.

If I could ever strive to be like someone, it would be my grandma. She was strong, freely expressed her opinions, and loved each family member like crazy. Dad wrote this poem about his mother (although I am not sure how the dress part and curly hair related to my dad! Perhaps it just rhymed).

Oh, mother dear, the years have passed,
And so gray has grown your hair.
Seems like yesterday, I was just a child,
And you so young and fair.

Time goes so fast, and now I'm grown,
And lines caress your face.
The years have surely swept us on,
So swift has been the race.

You dressed me in such pretty things,
And set curls in my hair.
But now you've grown older,
And it's my turn to show I care.

It seems so clumsy and hard at times,
To pay you all I owe.
Please forgive me, mother dear,
If how, I do not know.

Our blessed heavenly Father
has prepared a reward for you.
He has given your grandchildren
a mother who will do
The same pleasant and joyful things for them,
As a gift from us to you.

Grandpa

My grandpa was a hardworking man. He lost his prize herd of registered Holstein cows and one bull to Bang's disease around 1925; it took him years to recover from the loss. He had worked and saved money for years to buy this herd. Our grandma told the story of how, when grandpa got the news of the disease and experienced the subsequent loss of the entire herd, he sat down and cried.

It was like the end of his dream, the end of a way of life, so near and dear to his heart. For him, it was cataclysmic.

When grandpa couldn't farm, he worked on the railroad or in the creamery in town.

A stalwart tree my Dad to me
He has stood through storm and gale
When death and life
Knocked on our door
Our great tree did not fail
The roof upon our house was sound
And living there was good
Each day Dad brought the fixins home
So Mom could cook the food
A good and quiet man was he
Our guide throughout the years.
He was always there to share our joys
And dry away our tears.

I mentioned to Dad one day that he looked a lot like his dad. He told me, "Better to look like your own dad than someone else's dad." Dad could pop off those one-liners like a stand-up comedian.

Something was wrong with Grandpa. They moved from the country to a house in town, but ultimately my grandma couldn't take care of him. He was confused and becoming obstinate. My grandpa died the day before Thanksgiving in 1967 at age seventy-four. He had "hardening of the arteries," or as we call it now, dementia. In my last pictures of Grandpa he was lying in a hospital bed, oblivious to his surroundings.

A precious life stolen from our family by dementia. Did he have Lewy body dementia? We will never know. I was only nine when Grandpa died, but I have a few good memories of being on the farm with him. We would always laugh when he removed his false teeth and make a face, and he stood up for me when my sister tricked me into taking a bite of a wax apple!

Dad further wrote about his dad as follows:

Cold and bleak the winter night,
His grave I could not see.
They had tamped the earth and smoothed the sod
And hid it all from me.
Had my father really lived and been buried that very day?
Or was it all a dream to me, that would not go away?
Were all the years he lived and worked,
Lived and worked in vain?

Wasn't it just a fresh-filled grave, and was there not a gain?
I think of the creamery and the railroad shop,
And so many years of toil.
And best of all, he loved the farm,
And working in the soil.
But farther on and closer still,
Whether steel track or sod,
I find the better memory is
He gave first place to God.

A Soldier

If the bleakness of the Great Depression formed Dad, World War II molded his outlook on life. On March 5, 1945, at age eighteen, he eagerly joined the Navy, hoping to connect with the troops overseas to beat the Nazis and fascists. Finishing high school was trivial next to this greater ambition.

Dad spent his Navy years at the U.S. Naval Station in Norfolk, Virginia, where he earned the rank of coxswain. The coxswain oversees the navigation and steering in a small boat. Their main task is to ensure the others in the boat are safe.

Coxswain is a good description of how my dad lived his life during and post-Navy. I think he would have liked to run his home like a naval instructor; however, I'm sure he discovered raising four daughters had a whole different spin!

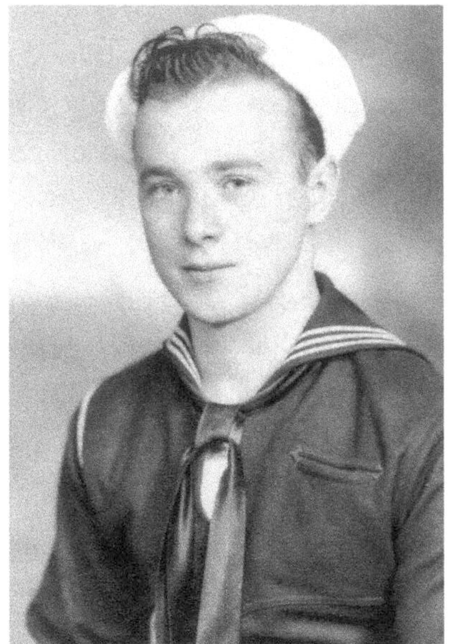

Navy Man

Much to his disappointment, the war ended before Dad had a chance to go overseas. On October 31, 1946, Dad received an honorable discharge and a medal called "Victory World War II, American Area." He also received this general commendation:

Lee Eggerud
Coxswain
U.S. Navy

To you who answered the call of your country and served in its Armed Forces to bring about the total defeat of the enemy, I extend the heartfelt thanks of a grateful Nation. As one of the Nation's finest, you undertook the most severe task one can be called upon to perform. Because you demonstrated the fortitude, resourcefulness and calm judgment necessary to carry out that task, we now look to you for leadership and example in further exalting our country in peace.

Harry S. Truman

Dad, like many men and women of that era, answered the call of duty in World War II. Fortitude, resourcefulness, and calm judgment—these qualities described Dad when times were tough. Maybe it even helped him deal with Lewy many years later.

Ever the poet and patriot, Dad wrote this poem called "Unknown, and Yet"

O, soldier boy, how did you die
as 'neath the cross of stone you lie?
A mother's boy known only to God,
who rests beneath the grassy sod,
crying out, "What was my life, only war and bitter strife?
Once the better things I knew,
to walk and feel the morning dew.
The scent of flowers filled the air,

I made bouquets for my girl's hair
and loved and worked for my native land.

When called, I offered up my hand.
We'll turn the enemy from our shore
and our land will be free forevermore.
Some will not return and shall surely die
but I knew, somehow, it would not be.
I said, "I shall return, and a hero be.
My fairest love that day I'll see."
But alas, this dream shall never be
No more the sunlight shall I see,
nor feel the cool breeze blow around,
nor see flowers grow from out the ground.

A mother's son with bleeding breast,
dying, unknown, gone to rest.
So if today our land be free,
and partly so because of me,
my life and death are not in vain—
for those I love there is a gain.
Now as you live and love in this land made free,
sometimes, please stop and think of me.

Chapter 3

Family Years

Today come go for a walk with me
Among the flowers fair
We'll stroll among the lilies
And along the river where
We can build a house of memories
Of our talks and things we do
Because life is always pleasant
When I'm building days with you,
The bricks we build the walls from
Are the experiences we share
The mortar is the love that comes
When people really care.
Houses of memories are never finished

They go on from year to year,
Sometimes through our laughter
And sometimes with a tear.

Caring for His Own

In 1945 there was hustle and bustle everywhere. Men returning from war, women leaving wartime jobs to become housewives. Everyone was looking for the new American dream.

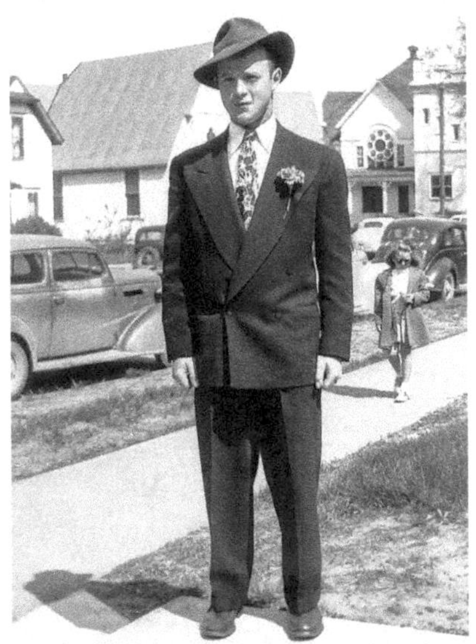

Dad as a Young Man

My parents were both living in Minneapolis; Dad was working, and Mom was going to business school to be a bookkeeper. They met on the steps of a bus as the seats were all taken.

Love blossomed. Dad promised Mom if she married him "she would always have her own washer and dryer," likely a big selling point in the 1940s!

He also told her the two scars on either side of his neck were war wounds from a bayonet that pierced his neck. (They were a result of neck drainage tubes from a childhood disease.) Imagine his embarrassment when he had to confess the truth to his future in-laws.

They were married by my grandfather, a minister, in Iowa in 1947.

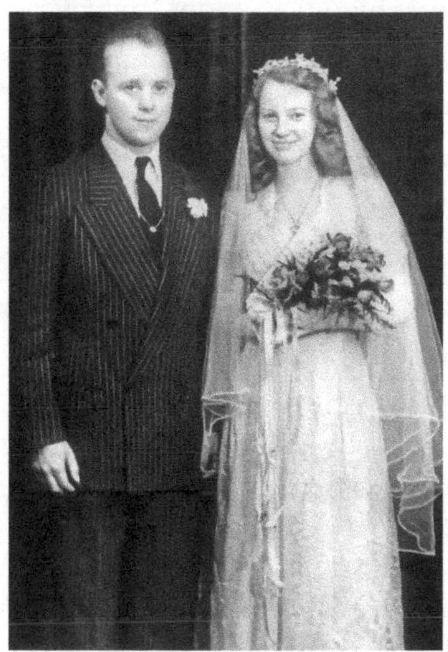

Mom and Dad's Wedding Day

Over the years my parents bought two different suburban homes, had four daughters, one dog, and several station wagons. Dad was fiercely independent, physically strong, and was making his way in life. His early years of working on the farm, selling papers, and joining the Navy had molded his character.

Dad had this Bible verse highlighted in his Bible: "*But if any provide not for his own, and especially for those of his own house, he hath denied this faith, and is worse than an infide*l." 1 Timothy 5:8, KJV.

This verse reflected his belief system that governed much of his life. In later years, I became baffled by an apparent change in his outlook, when he abandoned his traditional business and barely made a living.

Even though my father did not finish high school, he was ambitious and smart. (He was awarded his General Education Diploma or GED while in the Navy.) For many years Dad ran a ceiling tile business, bidding on jobs, managing a crew, and supporting his family. He named the company "Continental Sound Control."

On family trips, Dad would spot a building under construction.

Brake the car!

"Wait here!" he said as he ran into the building. A few minutes later he'd jump back in the car waving a piece of paper, announcing he had successfully lined up another ceiling tile job.

On vacations to Seattle or California to visit family, we would go and come home in a week. At every stop he would call back to "the business" to ensure things were running smoothly in his absence.

Dad set ceiling tile in many buildings in Minnesota and neighboring states. We would stop at a restaurant for lunch, or at a medical clinic or a church where he would proclaim, "I did the ceilings here." Often in a building he would look up to examine the ceiling job. He knew exactly when the tile was straight or a little mismatched. He would never be verbally critical, but he would frown a bit whenever he saw an old ceiling that could use his handiwork. Sometimes he would talk to the owner and lo and behold—he would land another job!

If he saw a ceiling needing repair, it would be an opportunity to bid for a repair job.

As a young girl I adored going to the construction jobs with Dad. I'd pick up little metal "slugs" off the floor, which were punch-outs from electrical boxes. I fancied they were money as they were about the size of nickels. I'd skip around the scaffolds,

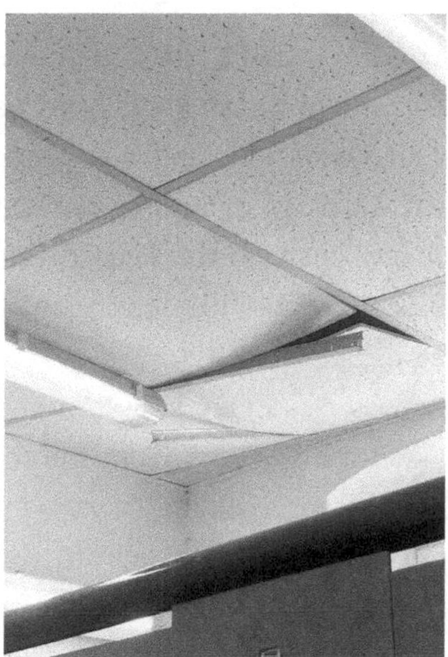

Repair Needed

oblivious to the electricians, plumbers, and painters. (I'm certain my father kept an eye on me to make sure I was safe.) To this day I get nostalgic when I see construction workers.

When the Billy Graham Association came to Minneapolis, Dad's company was the selected ceiling tile contractor, and he took me to visit Dr. Graham's new office. One of Dad's favorite stories was about Billy Graham and me. No, I never met Dr. Graham, but as Dad said, "Nancy's claim to fame is she used Billy Graham's toilet before him!" When he was getting older and forgetful, this was one story he would remember—and always laughed at his own humor!

Now that's an uffda!

Dad had a great business partner who worked tirelessly alongside him for years. For a while he had up to a dozen workers.

Dad loved to teach people the ceiling tile trade. Much to my mother's chagrin, at times Dad hired down-and-out folks—a man who drank too much or a friend's son who, in desperation, robbed a bank, served his time, and was released from jail. He would give a chance to almost anyone without a second thought. He hired students from the local Christian college or a friend of a friend who needed a job. When my husband was laid off Dad gave him work, and he started his nephew, another son-in-law, and others in the tile-setting profession.

To me, the business was everything to him. He worked hard, long hours to provide for his ever-growing family.

"Vacation! You're taking vacation!" Dad would scold me after I entered the workforce and took a day off. As a self-employed person, not working meant you were not making money. (Or maybe it just meant he wasn't in control!) Work was the end-all and be-all to this man of the Greatest Generation.

It is important that you understand my dad, so you can appreciate the impact of Lewy. This self-made man overcame his Depression-era childhood to run a business and raise a family. When he wasn't calculating a ceiling tile job on the back of a napkin, he was writing poetry or sharing a pie break with his family or friends.

My dear and precious little one
You know I love you so.
But there is One who loves you
More than I, you know.
He who bled and died for you,
Of whom all heaven sings,
'Tis He who comes to you today,
With healing in His wings.

A Man and His Treasures

He was the daddy of four daughters. I have a picture he gave each of us as adults. We four sisters had surrounded him in a restaurant, no doubt out for pie (he loved pie); Dad was pleased as could be. He attached a little note to each of the framed pictures, "A man and his treasures." (I'd show it to you, however I was having a bad hair day that decade.)

First came Sister 1, born nine months to the day after my parents were married. Three years later, along came Sister 2. Two girls, a perfect family.

They were surprised when seven years later I came on the scene! An "old age" child, they lamented at age thirty.

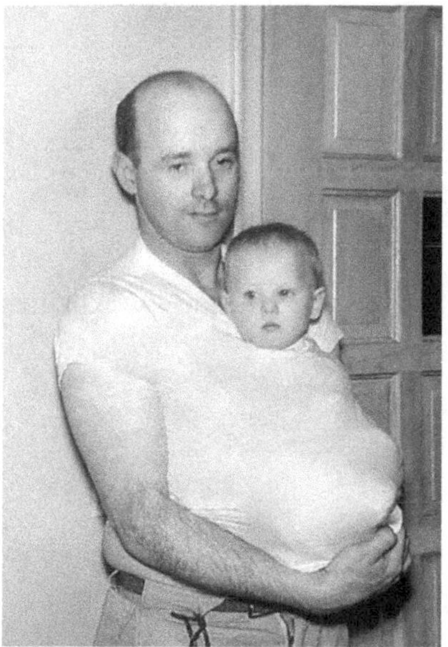

Dad Holding Me

Then came an even bigger surprise seven years after me, Sister 4. There were seventeen years between Sister 1 and Sister 4.

We waited anxiously until Dad came home from work each day. From time to time, he worked out of town, once for a very long stretch in North Dakota. The house lit up when he came back to his girls. He always sent us postcards when he was out of town for a stretch.

He wrote to me:

Hi Nancy,

Just thought I'd drop you a line.

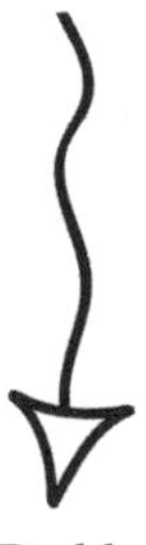

Love, Daddy

Or he would use one of the many nicknames he came up with for us:

Hi Lulu,

How is my girl today? No kiss last nite or this morning, and no faces either. I wondered if that other tooth came through last night? You and Mama kiss each other for Daddy.
I love you, sweetie.

Dad

Dad was a joke teller and always loved humor. Here he is "playing" checkers with our dog, Melody.

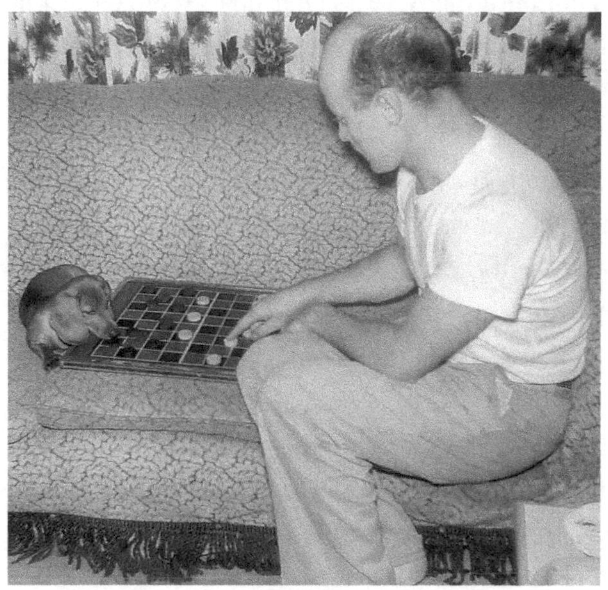

Checkers

There was never any physical discipline from Dad; all he had to do was give us "the look" of disappointment, and we wilted.

Living his Christianity was very important to Dad. No matter how busy he was, he made sure his daughters went to church. We attended Sunday mornings, Sunday evenings, and youth group on Wednesdays.

Dad's love for his family and for people was second to his love for God, and he made certain we understood and appreciated our Creator. He taught Sunday school, collected the offering, and met with small groups of men from church for pie and coffee. Serving the church was second nature to him.

Another favorite verse highlighted in his Bible was: "*Give, an d it shall be given unto you; good measure, pressed down, shaken together, and running over, shall men give into your bosom. For with the same measure that ye mete withal it shall be measured to you again*" (Luke 6:38, KJV).

It was not until many years later that I realized just how generous our dad was to people.

The Annoying Father

Unfortunately, he did not stay such a nice guy. Out of the blue he became very annoying. This coincidentally happened when I was an adolescent.

As a child, I was amazed by him, but as an adolescent "Father" became quite annoying. He would say, "Why are you never home so I can see you?"

And I would think, "Why are you always working and not home?"

But I wouldn't dare verbalize my thoughts; I'm not sure if it was fear, respect, or because I internalized my feelings. This I know; we girls did not "talk back."

For many years I was certain my birth was bad timing in his life. I heard stories of how he adored and played with Sister 1 and Sister 2. By the time I came along, he was just a serious workaholic (in my view).

Then cute little "Sister 4" was born seven years after me, the joy of my parent's "old age" (they were all of thirty-nine). Everyone adored the little cute blond girl. (Except for me from time to time. The only time I ever remember my mother hitting me was when she slapped me for calling my baby sister "a brat.")

They say middle children often feel excluded and lost. The oldest child receives more responsibility and privileges, and the youngest is indulged. In some ways I was a classic middle child, although as time went on, I took on many traits of an oldest child, as there were so many years between my older sisters and me.

As an adolescent, Dad and I were aliens. Or more accurately, *he* was an alien! The Alien Dad.

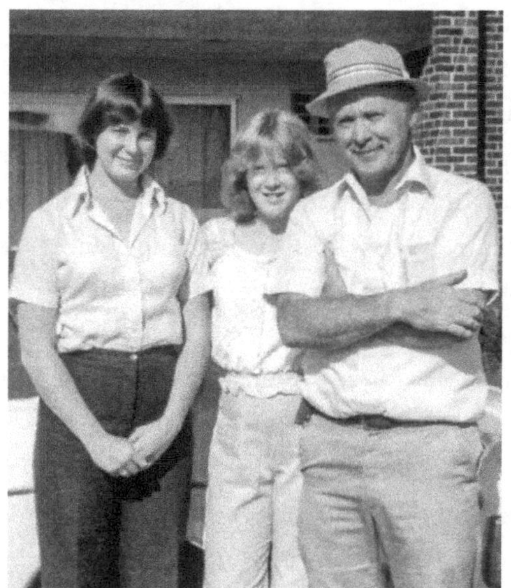

Me, my Sister and the Alien Dad

Where he was outgoing, I was shy. I liked my room messy; he threatened to take the door off and fill pillowcases with my stuff. (Ironically, years later, I was much more organized, and he and his stuff became scattered. Maybe due to Lewy?)

I liked to sleep in; he wired a speaker into my bedroom and blasted "Chicken Fat" into my tired ears on Saturday mornings. Go to You Tube and listen to "Chicken Fat" to get the full effect of how annoying a father could be.

Even though he was the son of a strong mother, the brother of four amazing sisters, and the father of four daughters, I deemed him to be quite sexist (common in his generation). "Those women-libbers" he would say.

Rosalyn Carter, wife of Jimmy Carter—my goodness, she sat in the Cabinet meetings and tried to run the country.

Gloria Steinem, the personification of the breakdown of the moral fiber of this country.

I, on the other hand, embraced women's rights at an early age. My favorite song: "I am Woman [hear me roar]" sung by Helen Reddy. (Again, a great YouTube listen.)

He discovered my Helen Reddy record that not only contained "I am Woman," but also "I don't Know How to Love Him" from "Jesus Christ Superstar." "Jesus Christ Superstar" was sacrilegious in Dad's worldview. So he threw out my favorite record—that made me super mad!

Talk about sex—oh, no—that was off limits! His only advice about sex was, "I know how men think!" when he didn't approve of a dress I wore.

Of course, he never told me how men think.

I've been married more than thirty-eight years and have two adult sons. I have a clue how men think, at least about *that* topic. But really, Dad, it would have been helpful to have a little more detail! (Hint to you dads out there.)

Despite his talk, he was never outwardly demeaning to women in their presence, and seemed to revere females. There was one woman he especially thought about highly.

Who's that lady sewing that cloth?
She says her name is Betsy Ross.
I said, "What are you doing with that old rag?"
She said, "Can't you see? I'm sewing a flag!"
"Who told you to do a thing like that?"
Says she, "A fella named George in a funny hat."
"Where did he come from, this guy named George?"
"He came in half froze from Valley Forge.

I know it sounds like a mystery,
But George said me and the flag
Would go down in history."
And sure enough, it was no lie,
'Cause here we are on the Fourth
of July.

The Good Times

We had great family times: trips to visit grandparents, aunts and uncles, and cousins.

My mom made holidays and birthdays special, creating our own special birthday cake and making all sorts of cookies for Christmas. Much of this came from her Swedish heritage. (The Swedes are a lot like the Norwegians; however, Swedes love sugar; Norwegians love cream. A wonderful combination, of course. I'd like to think I have the best of both heritages.)

The best treat of all was the lefse-making tradition. Every Thanksgiving and Christmas Dad would mix the potatoes, cream, and butter, get out the big round grills, and make the traditional big round lefse.

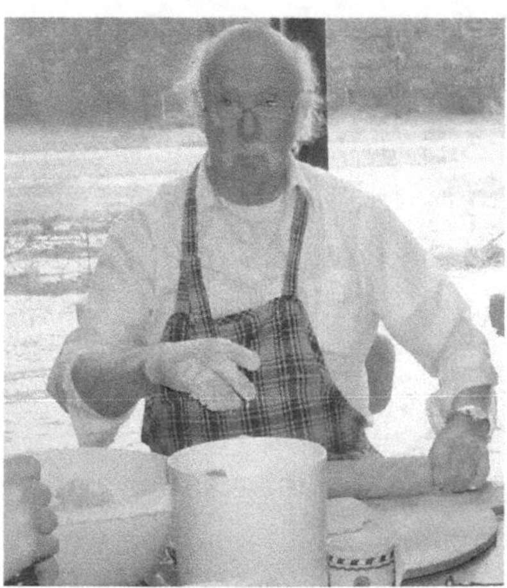

Making Lefse

Everyone loved giving and receiving gifts. They were literally piled high around the Christmas tree, as stated in this poem.

Gifts are piled high today beneath the Christmas tree,
Many bright and happy things
for everyone to see.
Things bought down at the store,
made so far away,
Taken home and wrapped,
to be exchanged on Christmas Day.

But you know the ones I love the most,
the very best you'll find,
Are made with loving, caring hands,
and a heart so gentle and kind.
Each and every separate thing
is handled and formed with care,

Touched by those very loving hands,
who have happiness to share.
So with special thanks this poem goes out
to such a one as this,
That took the time and cared enough,
to share their own Christmas.

Along with the lefse, my other best Christmas memory is Dad reading the Christmas story out of the Bible on Christmas Eve. As young kids, we would be antsy sitting through the story, as we couldn't open gifts until he had read the story! Now I look back with great nostalgia, wishing I could hear Dad's voice share the

Good News in Luke 2. Here it is in the King James Version, which is the version we used as I was growing up.

> *"And it came to pass in those days, that there went out a decree from Caesar Augustus that all the world should be taxed. (And this taxing was first made when Cyrenius was governor of Syria.) And all went to be taxed, everyone into his own city.*
>
> *"And Joseph also went up from Galilee, out of the city of Nazareth, into Judaea, unto the city of David, which is called Bethlehem; (because he was of the house and lineage of David). To be taxed with Mary his espoused wife, being great with child.*
>
> *"And so it was, that, while they were there, the days were accomplished that she should be delivered. And she brought forth her firstborn son, and wrapped him in swaddling clothes, and laid him in a manger, because there was no room for them in the inn.*
>
> *"And there were in the same country shepherds abiding in the field, keeping watch over their flock by night. And, lo, the angel of the Lord came upon them, and the glory of the Lord shone round about them: and they were sore afraid. And the angel said unto them, Fear not: for, behold, I bring you good tidings of great joy, which shall be to all people.*
>
> *"For unto you is born this day in the city of David a Savior, which is Christ the Lord. And this shall be a sign unto you; Ye shall find the babe wrapped in swaddling clothes, lying in a manger.*
>
> *"And suddenly there was with the angel a multitude of the heavenly host praising God, and saying, Glory to God in the highest, and on earth peace, good will toward men.*
>
> *"And it came to pass, as the angels were gone away from them into heaven, the shepherds said one to another, let us now go even unto Bethlehem, and see this thing, which is come to pass, which the Lord hath made known unto us.*

And they came with haste, and found Mary, and Joseph, and the babe lying in a manger.
"And when they had seen it, they made known abroad the saying which was told them concerning this child. And all they that heard it wondered at those things which were told them by the shepherds.
"But Mary kept all these things and pondered them in her heart. And the shepherds returned, glorifying and praising God for all the things that they had heard and seen, as it was told unto them" (Luke 2:19 KJV).

Many years later I had the privilege of visiting Bethlehem in the West Bank of Israel. I saw Shepherds' Field, where the shepherds heard the Good News of Jesus' birth. I also visited the Church of the Nativity, where Jesus was possibly born. I cried at the Nativity. How Dad would have loved to visit those holy sites!

A More Normal Dad

Dad started to act more like a normal human being as I got older. By the time I went to college in St. Paul, not far from home, we were able to have a conversation again without one of us (primarily me) becoming irritated. Dad would be the first one I'd call when I had a flat tire (and I had a lot of them because he kept finding me retread tires for my car). He would swing by for a piece of pie or cup of coffee when he was in my neighborhood.

I waitressed for several years, but grew tired of the sexist, demeaning environment in two different restaurants. When I could no longer tolerate waitressing, he hired me "on the job", which meant I went to construction jobs with him. I put up ceiling tile or clean up after the workers. This, however, was frowned upon by the union as I didn't carry a union card, so my career in construction did not last long. (Which was just as well, I did not like the noisy, dusty environment.)

Dad and I grew closer, but always you could find a push-pull element in our father-daughter relationship. We never exactly waltzed in harmony; our dancing was more like the bunny-hop—we could be in the same line but still do our own moves.

Chapter 4

Changes

Dad branched out in his fifties. Now having successfully graduated from my fifties, I get it—life can start to look different as we age. Is there more to life? Are we mere mortals? How do we live our earthly dreams before it's too late?

We were surprised to discover this man with rough hands, who prided himself on arm-wrestling down any of his sons-in-law, could do fine artwork.

Dad took on some interesting hobbies, one being cake decorating. Upon taking a community ed class, he would practice his new-found talent on family members. It reminds me of my aunt's story of a family muffin-baking time. She said "Lee was great at making muffins. I couldn't understand, at first, why his were better than mine. My mother explained it. She said, 'He has a gentler hand.' In other words, he didn't beat the batter to death as one had to do for a successful cake."

I do not recall too many fancy cakes, however, after the initial decorating frenzy subsided.

Calligraphy, on the other hand, was an art form he could embrace. (I thought it was an interesting hobby for a guy with such bad handwriting. I too have bad handwriting and did not share his passion, or his patience, to make those decorative characters.)

Perhaps the calligraphy led to one of his favorite side jobs, making hand-carved wooden signs. He carefully picked out the correct wood for his projects, carved the letters, and varnished the signs, often in multiple shades.

Clowning Around

Wearing a big red nose and a clown suit became one of Dad's favorite pastimes. He and a couple of friends joined a clowning club. Dad would dress up for the grandkids' birthdays, march in parades, or entertain kids at parties. He could be such a fun dad and grandpa!

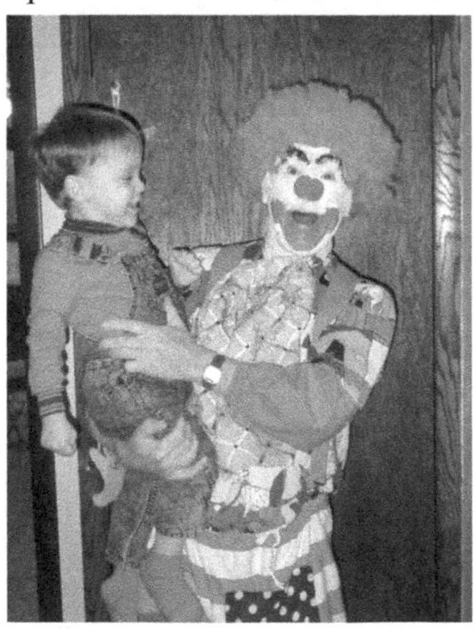

Dad with Grandson Corey

The circus came to town back in my dad's young days in Brainerd. The paperboys would watch them unload, and the elephants were always used to push and pull the wagons. They would grunt and snarl and growl in their cages. Dad's older brother would try to get jobs with the circus so he could get free tickets to bring his younger siblings; often they would succeed. Maybe this is where Dad first saw circus clowns and determined that could be him someday.

Glass Grinding and Crystal Repair

Another side gig caught Dad's interest—glass grinding and crystal repair. He had been in contact with a gentleman in Florida with a flourishing repair business. With extra frequent flyer miles, I acquired a round trip ticket for him to fly to Florida and learn how to fix delicate crystal, china, and glass.

Perhaps that is when he wrote this poem:

The plane piercing through the sky,
Clouds so fluffy floating by.
What river is that flowing free,
Past the mountains to the sea?
Too small to ever catch the eye,
Are all the people passing by?
Hurrying, scurrying everywhere,
Can't be seen, but surely there.

Glass grinding and crystal and china repair turned out to be a great business for our dad; it brought out the artist in him. For many years he traveled from town to town, advertising his craft. People would come from miles around to have their treasures fixed. His glass-grinding business was featured in both a magazine and a newspaper.

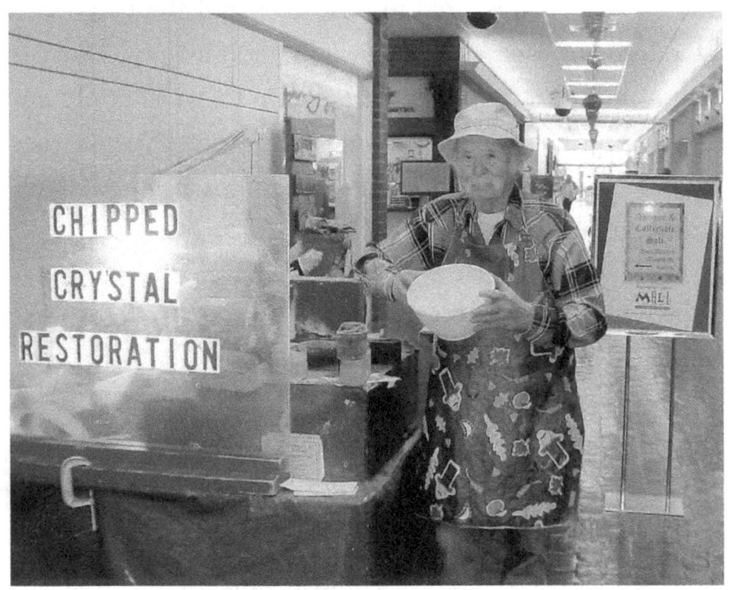

Making the Broken New Again

Later in life he thanked me again for that free airplane ticket, saying, "You helped me earn a living for many years." I was pleased I could be a part of bringing him so much joy and a source of income.

However, I didn't anticipate one move on his part that would cause me personal heartache for years.

Slippery Slope

Dad was still running the tile business (the real bread-and-butter work), but he increasingly lost his motivation for construction work. As a result, I believe some of his business practices suffered.

I didn't always approve of his business or personal ventures. He borrowed money from people, including my husband and me, and then seemed to squander the funds. He'd swap money from one bank account to the next to stay afloat and kept borrowing against the house. I wasn't thrilled about some of his friends and colleagues.

You may wonder why my husband and I lent him money. It was for mini-donut equipment, one of his great side ventures. We wanted to keep believing in him. I'm pretty sure he forgot he owed us money. My husband also "gave" my dad a truck. It seems Dad also forgot he was going to pay us for the truck. We always felt sorry for him because as he got older, he clearly did not make the money he had made when the tile business was going strong.

Do people really change that much in their fifties?

Talk about push-pull, my mother and father were *very* different. My mother was introverted, loved to stay at home and read or do household chores, and spent time with a few special friends. She was the ultimate housewife and mom, making all our favorite foods and doing crafts with us when we were little. She was the bookkeeper for my dad's business for years and poured her whole heart into the task.

I believe she suffered from depression and did not handle stress well.

Dad was extroverted, and he loved to travel and make friends with everyone. He was very even-keel emotionally, and I think her sadness mystified him.

At one point in his early fifties, Dad moved out of the house, leaving my mother behind. I became my mother's confidant and emotional caretaker. Even though I was at college and working many hours a week to support myself, I called her every day.

I will never know what happened behind the scenes between my parents, and I do not want to know.

This is hard for me to tell, as I don't want to degrade either of their characters or memories. There were mitigating factors, but I had a hard time forgiving my dad. My heart became hard, and I lost a lot of trust in my father.

Here is a rather depressing poem Dad wrote during that season of his life. (Most of his poetry wasn't dated, but this one contained the year.)

The horse stood at the starting gate,
Chomping at the bit.
He had a dream of a winning race,
And thought that this was it.
He had lost and tried,
And won, as many as he could.
He wanted life to be a winning race,
As anybody would.

But treatment cruel, and lack of food
And water took its toll.
One day he knew that death would come,
Before he'd reach his goal.

Bit by bit the dying came,
And soon the spirit fled.
And in the stable cold and dark,
They found the great horse dead.

In tears and shock the owner said,
"This thing cannot be.
With hay and grain and loving care,

You'll race again for me.
What I did was all for love,
And you know I really care."
So he brought the better things he had,
And spoke with words so fair.

But in life and marriage, as with racing horses,
Death is the final word.
And all the tender loving care,
And pretty words cannot be heard.

So if little by little, and year by year,
You extinguish love's sweet flame,
It won't be there to warm you,
When you're ready to play the game.

His behavior also left me confused—was he not supposed to be a Christian? Aren't parents supposed to model upstanding behavior? How could he do this to my mom! How could he do it to me and my younger sister, who still lived at home? I was at the cusp of adulthood, but that didn't matter—I was still Daddy's little girl inside.

The Bible tells us God is the judge of others, not us. However, I imagined myself an excellent judge; it was way too easy to occupy that judgment seat myself. I have prayed for forgiveness for my lack of understanding and rush to judgment.

Eight months later Dad moved back; my parents must have come to some sort of understanding.

But back to Dad and me—there were a lot of missteps in our dancing in those years. I was sure he was stepping on my toes on purpose.

Now I wonder, was Lewy already creeping in? Was his brain changing even in his fifties and sixties? Was he in mid-life crisis, male menopause? Was he tempted, making bad choices? And why did I imagine myself the judge of his decisions?

Dad was still his hardworking and humorous self, and people adored him.

Life went on; through the next decade I was busy with work, family, volunteering, and not paying a lot of attention to what was happening with Dad. Little did I know what was ahead. But before we start talking about my nemesis, Lewy, here is another side of Dad's humor.

Dad had an aversion to being overweight and often referred to himself as the "Thin, Trim Dad."

My all-time favorite poem:

I wanted to be so slim and trim
As anyone would be
Growing ever more beautiful
For everyone to see.
So I dieted and exercised, and I really, really tried.
I brutalized my body, until I nearly died.
Just to be so gorgeous, sensual and slinky;
But darn the luck—look at me now:
Done in by a twinky.

Another one of his claims was "I am the germ-free dad." Perhaps it was to assure my mother he wouldn't pass germs on to us kids. And maybe it was true, he was seldom ill.

Even odder behavior surfaced in Dad's late sixties and early seventies. He was easily distracted and lost his enthusiasm for "the business," barely making enough money to survive. He lost tools, jackets, and workers.

Conversely, he said he would never stop working. "I don't have to save for retirement. I'll always work." Smile. Snicker.

I do not know when his brain changes began. I follow people on social media who are now diagnosed with Lewy body dementia in their fifties and sixties. I wish I had answers, and I hope science can find ways to diagnose and treat these diseases sooner.

Chapter 5

Dementia Creeps In

Dad was in his seventies when his dementia and I collided. It is when our dance with Lewy began, although Lewy was nameless and faceless for years.

By 2005, it was clear there was an elephant in the room. Dad was almost eighty, I was fifty. Aside from his memory problems and glaucoma, he was in excellent physical health. Dad was still strong as an ox, but he suffered from dizziness. In those days, there were no sides on the scaffolds. He fell off the scaffolds a couple of times, and due to his good balance or the grace of God, landed on his feet. But with the onset of dizziness, he gave up the scaffold climbing and the ceiling tile business for good.

My three sisters and I consulted regularly, what to do? Was this just aging, or was there something seriously wrong with him? It came to a head one day when he called me to meet for lunch.

Dad was still driving. His office, two rooms rented in the bottom of an old building in northeast Minneapolis, was only a few miles from where I worked. Over the years, Dad had several offices, but I am certain this was his favorite.

Can You Help?

From time to time, Dad and I met for lunch. Everyone knew him by name in the Thai restaurant between our two offices. This day, however, he wanted to meet at a sandwich and soup shop.

As we stood in line, Dad looked at me, handed me his checkbook, and said, "I can't figure this out anymore. Can you help?"

Wow. This was a big step for my dad. He was always a very private person when it came to finances. My sisters and I never had any idea how much money he made, and as he aged, he kept his financial dealings away from my mother.

I knew my parents were having financial struggles, but I had no idea what was happening.

He asked me to help him, and being the task-orientated administrative daughter, I plunged right in.

I went to his office, set out a basket, and instructed him to place bills and other mail in the basket. I would stop by at least once a week and sort through his mail.

I dug and found out he had five bank accounts, all with minimal money. On top of the bank accounts, Dad had several credit cards; he took out cash from ATMs on those high-interest credit cards. Tardy payments resulted in late fees. Within a month of collecting his mail, I calculated he owed over $8,000 in outstanding bills.

(Maybe we should count ourselves fortunate; I know one family whose mom had accumulated $20,000 in debt in the early stages of Alzheimer's.)

My parents' income consisted of Dad's Social Security, which he gave my mother to pay the household bills with, and Mom's minimal Social Security. Then there was his "work," which consisted of the crystal repair business, selling mini-donuts, and making wooden signs for people (which he often gave away).

I was horrified. What to do? How would they get out of this mess?

What Will Mom Say?

To understand where my father was at this point, you need a little understanding of my mother (whom I fondly called "Little Mother," as I had quickly bypassed her in height by age thirteen). As I mentioned, Little Mother was introverted, had not worked out of the home since before she was married, and undoubtedly suffered from depression. As we were growing up, she often had physical illness and pain, and she had multiple surgeries.

Raised by a loving but poor ministerial family, in her adult years Little Mother carefully accounted for every cent. Her checkbook was manually balanced to the penny. A perfectionist, she kept the books for Dad's business for years, and certainly contributed to his business success. She hated debt, and in later years was appalled at loans my dad took out to fund his business.

Some years before this, he decided she did not need to keep the books anymore. I suppose the ceiling tile business was not bringing in much money anymore, so he handled his little side businesses on his own or with other helpers.

Now I was faced with how to handle Dad's accumulating debt.

I talked to my sisters, prayed, and explored alternatives. The best temporary solution we could come up with was for my parents to take a loan against the house.

I planned a meeting with my parents. The three of us gathered around their brown Formica kitchen table, the one that had been there since my childhood. The table had a little red spot, a defect that always bugged me. I stared at the red spot, wondering where to start. This ranked as our worst parental moments to date, but not of those we would experience in the future.

I slowly explained the situation to Mom—how Dad had spent on the credit cards and how little income his "business" generated. I included the fact he had to pay rent and phone bills for his office.

Dad sat there silent, already with a blank stare in his eyes.

Mother cried, abhorring the thought of taking out more debt on the house at their ages.

I was sick to my stomach. This was truly the last place I wanted to be, sitting at the brown kitchen table with the two of them, talking about money.

Would she agree? What would happen to them? Where would they live? How could they live?

I did not realize it at the time, but this is one point where my faith in God's provision was sorely tested.

It was also a time I clearly heard His voice. "I will take care of their finances. They will be okay." Did I hear an audible voice, like Moses with the burning bush? No. It was a whisper in my ears and my heart, and just like Moses, I knew it was the voice of the Almighty. In the coming years, I clung to that promise.

Come morning, with your rising sun,
And overcoming light,

The worries and fears that grip my heart
Seem then to take their flight.
Each day that's new gives promise
Of a chance to overcome
God's not author of this fear
That makes His children run.

O morning light and precious day,
A promise to every heart.
This is the time, the night is spent,
It's time to make your start.
So hold your promise, take that step,
Reach out your hand anew.
Fear will leave when hope is born
That winner will be you.

My mother agreed to take out the house loan. None of us knew the future, but at least they were covered for the moment. We paid off the credit cards, which I promptly put into safekeeping, and put Dad on an allowance.

That went over very well with Dad.

Not!

What to Do?

I paid his office bills; he continued to make a little money selling his wares. My mother paid the house bills out of their Social Security checks.

The bills were barely covered, the house needed repairs, and there was no money to spare. The logical conclusion was for them to sell the house.

It was also a matter of safety. Mom had severe osteoporosis. Hunched over with back pain, she could not safely go down the stairs to do the laundry or get food out of the freezer.

The situation continued to deteriorate.

The elephant in the room was getting bigger, consuming all our lives. My sisters and I knew we had to get Dad a diagnosis. God bless my sisters; they are three amazing, strong women. We each had a role.

- Sister 1, the eldest one, lived southeast of the Twin Cities (Minneapolis/St. Paul). She is the sweetest, most loving person you will ever meet. Once when I woke up from major surgery, she was wiping my forehead with a cool cloth and had ice chips handy for my dry mouth. From cutting toenails, to putting on pain patches, to just listening to stories, she lovingly served my parents.
- Sister 2, the second eldest, lived in the eastern part of the United States. While she could not always be here to help, she was just a phone call away to offer support and encouragement. I called her our "Angel of Mercy" as she always flew home just when there was a major crisis, and the rest of us were at our wit's end. She had worked as a clinical therapist for people with head injuries, and she understood medical terms and tough decision-making.
- Then there's me, Sister 3, the pragmatist, administrator, filler out of government paperwork, tracker of finances—all those analytical tasks fell to me. The "family hero." Every family needs a hero; however, it is not such a great place to be if you cannot set reasonable boundaries. I internalize my feelings, which is also not so good. It comes out in other ways, as I was to discover.

- Sister 4, my youngest sister, is a mix of love and understanding, with outstanding organization skills. She fell into the role of managing, coaxing, and guiding our dad into some of the difficult decisions to come. She would run over to our parents' house with homemade soup or a pastry treat.

I love all my sisters; they are truly my best female friends.

I am grateful we were able to work together on my parents' care. I grieve for families who cannot get along or have major caretaking disagreements. If this is your struggle, my advice is life is short, try to find ways to get along, or at least try to divvy up the caretaking duties for the sake of your loved ones.

My father had found his own doctor, a kind and highly intelligent physician specializing in gerontology. We saw him together several times. I'll call him Dr. S. Dad's main complaint was "dizziness," which can be a result of dementia. Dr. S recommended over-the-counter remedies.

Symptoms and Signs

The family put our heads together and came up with a list of symptoms. The following are notes given to Dr. S in December 2005.

Changes we have noticed in our father's daily activities:

- He is dizzy in the mornings and frustrated none of his doctor visits have addressed this or helped to alleviate the dizziness.
- Unhappy about all the doctor appointments and his family's involvement with his healthcare. Has been uncharacteristically snappy toward us about it.
- His driving has been affected (especially the last two years); drives very slowly. He has had several "mini accidents," such as brushing the sides of cars. He weaves in and out of

traffic and has been stopped and questioned about whether he's been drinking.

- Has become a very restless sleeper.
- Noticeably disoriented in unfamiliar settings, for example, on a family trip or at a family house for the holidays.
- During his birthday in November, and at Christmas, we noticed opening gifts was mechanically difficult.
- He cut a block of cheese with the dull side of the knife.
- He could not put a flashlight back together.
- He likes a bowl of milk, brown sugar and rice, a traditional Norwegian dish. When the rice was served on a plate, he poured milk over the rice.
- He asked what "percussion" is after hearing about his grandson's drum concert.
- He confuses which family member belongs to which family.
- On the positive side:
- He can recite poetry he's learned clearly.
- He can give directions clearly and in specific detail.

I learned it is important to be as specific as possible with symptoms and behavioral issues as it assists the medical team with a diagnosis.

Now that I know more about Lewy body dementia, many of these symptoms my dad exhibited seem like classic Lewy. However, hindsight is 20/20 and this was over a dozen years ago. If Dad developed Lewy body dementia now, would the medical community diagnose him sooner? Are doctors educated about the differences between Alzheimer's, Parkinson's, Lewy body dementia, vascular dementia, frontal lobe dementia—and all the others?

I am following a Facebook support group for caretakers of loved ones with Lewy body dementia. Many of these people are diagnosed at a younger age than my dad was. But Lewy continues to be unknown to many, and it's an insidious intruder into people's lives.

Dr. S, upon our request, scheduled an MRI, then referred us to a neurologist I'll call Dr. G. Sister 4 volunteered to take Dad to a series of appointments to obtain a diagnosis. Dr. G was kind and helpful, talking respectfully to our dad. Sister 4 was able to ask many questions and was able to call and talk to Dr. G directly for follow-up issues.

Part of the exam is a question-answer period, to be repeated to check for progression. It's called a mini-mental exam. Despite a caring medical team, the process is humiliating, especially to a man like Dad, a self-made businessman.

- Draw a clock.
- Who is the President?
- What month is this?
- Where do you live?

All are basic questions or tasks most of us could easily answer. But when dementia is knocking at the door, simple questions become frustrating and confusing. It made Dad frustrated and angry.

My father, however, was determined to beat the system. Once at the VA they gave him the "mini-mental" exam. He came out laughing, saying, "I showed that guy!" I asked how? He said, "That guy [the doctor] asked me 'Who is the President?' There was a picture of George Bush right behind him—and I got it right!"

You must appreciate humor when it comes.

The "Crazy" Disease

We waited anxiously for the diagnosis. Finally, a letter arrived. It seemed like relatively good news. He was diagnosed with a dementia "not in the pattern of Alzheimer's disease" called Vascular dementia.

Web MD states, "Vascular dementia happens when vessels that supply blood to the brain become blocked or narrowed. Strokes take place when the supply of blood carrying oxygen to the brain is suddenly cut off. However, not all people with stroke will develop vascular dementia.

Vascular dementia can happen over time as "silent" strokes pile up. Quite often, vascular dementia draws attention to itself only when the impact of so many strokes adds up to significant disability."[3]

Particularly affected was his "executive functioning".

Executive function is a set of mental skills that helps you get things done. These skills are controlled by an area of the brain called the frontal lobe. Executive function helps you:

- Manage time
- Pay attention
- Switch focus
- Plan and organize
- Remember[4]

Dad was *very* relieved. "At least I don't have 'that crazy disease.'" (Part of dementia is word-finding, and he couldn't recall "Alzheimer's," so he picked his own definition. No offense intended to any of my readers, but people with any sort of dementia are not "crazy"—it is a terrible label.)

Remember Ted Turner—He could not remember the names of the diseases either.

At times I have trouble recalling names of people or places. When it happens, I feel frustrated and embarrassed. How much more does this happen with full-blown dementia?

We felt we could deal with this diagnosis. Vascular dementia? A few mini strokes in the brain? Didn't sound so bad, if the strokes remained in the "mini" category. (Not to minimize vascular dementia, but I was ignorant at that time.)

If I were a ballerina, I would have danced a ballet.

Of course I didn't know what diagnosis would come much later, and he could well have had two brain diseases.

Chapter 6

The Storm

While we struggled to deal with our dad's dementia, we received bad news about our mom.

My mother's health was deteriorating, and she was in constant pain from a crumbling spine. Surgery was not an option; the only treatment was periodic steroid shots.

At age fifty-nine, Mom, a caregiver for her parents, had a small stroke. My parents did not have health insurance at the time, so she refused to go to the doctor. I of course did not hear about the stroke for a couple of days. Why worry us girls?

Fortunately, Mom had few side effects, although I noticed her ability to organize events took a down-turn.

After the stroke she was treated for high blood pressure. As she aged, she took multiple blood pressure medications that made her sleepy for several hours every morning. Trips to doctors increased for her, and we tried to take turns taking her. My husband, who got off work in the late afternoon, took her to several appointments, bless his heart.

Mom was in her early eighties when I took her to have an MRI on her back. We stopped at the grocery store, and when we got to the house and worked our way in, we heard the phone ring. Her physician was calling to say they found a tumor in her kidney. She was to see a specialty urologist as soon as possible.

I was shocked and heartbroken. There was not a lot of cancer in our family, but I wondered, "Was this the C word?" Not now, not for Mom, who lived the most wholesome life you could imagine.

I stayed long enough to tell my dad about my mom's kidney tumor when he got home. It was a rainy, dark Minnesota spring night. I drove the long way home on the side roads, tears falling down my cheeks the whole trip, listening to Christian radio. The song "Praise You In This Storm" by Casting Crowns came on, and I was struck by the words. The song talks about the rain, and the storm, and praising God despite the storm. (Go ahead and listen to it on YouTube to get the full message I received that night; I was unable to obtain a license to print the words here.)

As I drove through the rain, I was not certain that the message of the song applied to me.

- Praise God mother has cancer?
- Praise God dad has dementia?
- Praise God that their house is falling apart, and that they have no money?

My husband and I still had a very active teenage son, Corey, at home, along with an adult son. I worked full time at a stressful job requiring travel, and my husband had an hour drive to and from work each day. How could we deal with one more stressor in life?

Did the song really mean to praise God in *this* storm?

Ironically, coincidentally—or maybe by divine providence—"Praise You In This Storm" came on the radio periodically in the next several years when I needed it the most. I am still learning to "Praise Him In This Storm."

But that night I just cried in the rain all the way home.

Hallucinations

Mom had her left kidney removed, which required hospitalization and recovery in a care home.

This whole ordeal left our dad more confused. He began to get his wife mixed up with his mother, Ella. (The same Ella that pulled their ears when they wriggled in church from the itchy wool pants.) Several times when Mom was in the care home, Dad reported we were going to see his mother, or "Ma" as she was called. One time I was at their house and he called: "Hello? Is this Ma? I thought Ma was going to call!"

"No Dad, this is Nancy."

Around this time, he told us he saw an angel in the corner of his bedroom. Now I believe in angels. The Psalmist said:

"*For he will command his angels concerning you to guard you in all your ways; they will lift you up in their hands, so that you will not strike your foot against a stone*." (Psalm 91:11-12, NIV).

I also believe, as the Bible demonstrates, that people have seen angels from time to time. I'm not convinced my dad saw an angel that night, but who am I to say?

I do know he did not see me in the living room in a flowered dress, as he reported one day when I had not been near their house.

As we learned later, hallucinations are part of Lewy body dementia. But I didn't know about the signs and symptoms of Lewy body dementia; I just thought he was stressed and imagining things.

I just smiled and nodded, but inside I was scared. Why would vascular dementia cause so much confusion in his brain? We did not have the internet available in today's format, so we could not "google" signs and symptoms of the disease.

Mom spent a week recovering in a nursing home (her worst nightmare) and slowly recovered from her surgery.

Driving

Dad's old cargo Chevrolet van sat in the driveway. Brown, with white trim, showing its age. There was no back seat; instead it was filled with tools, pieces of wood, varnish, and scrunched-up clothes. Papers littered the floor, and should you decide to sit in the passenger seat, Dad would quickly move around stuff so there was room.

Do not sit in his van in your dress clothes, I quickly learned.

Most memorable about this van were the dents, nicks, and dings. And a few creases. I parked next to the old Chevy in my parents' driveway, cringing at a new crease on the side.

I walked in the door. The news on the TV was blaring.

"Dad, could you turn down the volume?"

"Yeah—where is that thing now?" (Finds the remote and turns down the TV volume.)

Dad loved to listen to the news, and this was the beginning of constant news, running all day.

"Did you know more soldiers were killed in that country over there today?"

"No, I did not."

"There was an earthquake in one of those island places."

"I didn't know, Dad; I've been at work all day."

"Dad, how did you get that new crease in the van?"

"That woman plowed right into me!" he replied. "I was pulling out of a parking lot and she drove right into my van!"

"Did you see her coming?"

Rather sheepishly he replied, "No, but she should be watching. Besides, everyone gets a few dings on their vehicles—it's just part of driving."

I shook my head.

We could never tackle the driving topic directly. That is not how Minnesotans handle controversy. Plus, I was the daughter; he was the father.

Dad had too much pride and independence to stop driving on his own.

I talked to my sisters; we agreed something had to be done. So as was my preferred method, I took the indirect route.

We had a doctor visit the next week. Dr. S sat at his little desk in the examining room. Dad sat next to him in a chair, and I sat on the other side of Dad, trying to remain inconspicuous.

Dr. S gave him his usual mini-mental exam. "What year is it?" "Summer" answered my dad. "Where do you live?" "At home." "What else is going on, Lee?" "I'm dizzy, and no one knows why!"

I pulled a sheet of paper out of my purse, scribbled "*DRIVING*" and held it up behind my dad's back. Dr. S said, "How is your driving going, Lee?" Surprised, Dad answered "Just fine." I rolled my eyes. "Well, good, let me know if you ever have a problem."

Dr. S ignored my glare.

The next month Dad had an eye doctor appointment. He regularly saw Dr. B due to progressive glaucoma. Surely Dr. B will pull him off the road, I thought. I conscripted the help of Sister 2 to help with a letter.

Together we drafted a letter to Dr. B, spelling out the driving issues and questioning Dad's ability to see, especially at night.

In the appendix you can find excerpts of various letters we wrote to health care providers and others regarding his health and driving.

Later, I asked Dad how the appointment went. "Fine, I like her a lot. She helps me see, and she really listens." That's it? I thought.

Later, when I accompanied Dad to another appointment, I caught up with Dr. B in the hall and asked her about the driving situation. Dr. B said if he could pass the eye exam at the license bureau, there was nothing she could do.

Clearly the medical community was not going to help with this problem. The sisters indirectly continued our quest to get him pulled off the road. (None of us wanted to be the culprit.)

Next step: write a letter to the Minnesota Department of Safety, the overseers of the drivers' bureau. Again, we explained the situation. Could they require a driver's test of him? They replied no; when his license expired, and he came in to get it renewed, they would determine if he could pass the eye test.

Dad had always been a law-abiding citizen. He would wave and chat with police officers. When I was growing up, one of my parents' closest friends was a former police officer I'll call Joe. As kids, we would often visit Joe's family. I'd play with their daughters, and the adults would chat.

Now the police became the enemy. We would pass a police car on the side of the road with the officer ticketing a driver. Dad would say, "Look at the police, ruining that poor guy's life."

Dad decided to drive to Brainerd but did not tell any of the daughters. Dad had driven to Brainerd hundreds of times and knew the route by heart. There was a certain split in the road, and the right-hand path leads to Brainerd.

Dad got confused, went left, then crossed the double white line to go right. An officer pulled him over and wrote him a ticket. On the back of the ticket the officer listed *five times* in the past year Dad had been pulled over but not ticketed.

The old Dad would not have shown me this ticket. This new Dad did not think of the consequences; out came the ticket for me to read to prove the police were out to "ruin his life."

Five warnings? Who gets five warnings?

Did those previous officers pull him over for weaving about the road and, happy he was not drinking, give him a warning? Perhaps they were charmed by his smile or that little chuckle. I do not know their reasoning.

I thought, "Why did they pull him over and *do nothing*?!"

Like he had done in the conversation about the dings on his van, he told me, "Everyone gets stopped by the police once in a while!" (I thought, not five times in one year; nor does everyone charm their way out of tickets like you!") I of course did not say this to him. That would have been too direct.

I did have a chat with his insurance agent, a nice man who recognized the problem. He said my parents' car insurance was going to go up, and we should think about taking Dad off the road.

Easier said than done, I explained to him.

At least there was a consequence this time. Dad received a letter from the state ordering him to retake the driver's test. (Did they connect the dots between our letter and the ticket? I will never know, but I would like to think the letter helped.)

This is it, we thought. He will never pass the test.

On his own, Dad went to the large driver's license testing facility. He tried to take the written test but could not figure out how to work the computer. He asked me to come with him the next time, so off we went to the driver's bureau together. Dad asked if I could help him take the test. They said no, he had to do it on his own, and he did not pass again.

He was told accommodations could be made for people who are unable to use computers.

Now Dad might have had brain processing issues, but he was still smart enough to figure out how to beat the system. He went to a smaller driver's bureau in our town. He asked for the accommodation, and one of the workers gave him the written test verbally. He told me, "The ladies were so excited I passed the test, they wanted to take me out to lunch!"

Seriously, does the whole world want this man, who is nearly unable to see at night and cannot read the driver's manual, loose on the highways?

And is there anyone on earth he can't charm?

Sister 1 and I decided to pay a visit to the local driver's bureau. (Good indirect way to address the issue.) We talked to the supervisor "Ralph." Ralph assured us he would personally give our dad the driving test and carefully assess his ability. Satisfied, certain our dad would not pass the actual driving test, we left the facility.

Guess what? He passed! Sister 1 and I went back to visit Ralph.

"How did he pass the test, Ralph?"

"Your dad did very well, no problems at all."

"Where did you drive with him?"

"Just right here in town, on the local roads."

"What about driving on the highway?"

"That isn't a requirement," said Ralph.

Seriously? Dad was still driving to his office in Minneapolis, which required driving on the highways daily.

What could we do? Nothing at this point, other than pray he didn't hurt himself or another person.

We will pick up on the driving saga later.

Chapter 7

A Big Decision

Thc year was 2007. As my mother was preparing for her kidney surgery, we realized we had to sell their house. It cost too much to keep up, repairs were needed—the windows were rotting, there was no hot water in the bathroom faucet, and it was falling into general disrepair.

Dad was paying the neighbor to mow the lawn. One day I was at the house when the neighbor came over and asked Dad for his $20 for lawn mowing. Dad paid him, and I am not saying thc man was doing anything questionable, but I did wonder if Dad would know if he paid him once a week or three times a week to mow.

My parents lived in the house for nearly fifty years. It was a three-bedroom rambler style made popular in the Midwest by the Greatest Generation. It was my father's pride; he built special shelving units and closets, built what we called "the breezeway," which was used as an office. The fixed-up basement had an extra bedroom, bathroom, and recreation room. (No egress windows where a person can easily climb out in case of fire were required back in those days.)

Our father would not even consider selling the house. He could be quite the stubborn Norwegian, and his daughters were certainly *not* going to tell him what to do. He was the man of the house, after all.

We suggested, cajoled, and sent our youngest sister over to coax him into selling the house. Not even she succeeded.

We tried to persuade Dad by telling him our mother could not safely live there anymore—she couldn't traverse the stairs to go to the basement to do the laundry. (We also reminded him about the squirrels that took up residence in the attic in the fall. The squirrels made my mom nuts (just a little pun).

No movement, not even a flinch on Dad's part. Clearly there was enough brain functioning to be firm on his house stance.

Minnesota does not have hurricanes or earthquakes. We remind ourselves of this in the cold, dark winters. Spring in Minnesota is beautiful.

Have you ever been in the garden
in the early days of spring?
When the flowers break forth from the earth,
and the robins begin to sing?

As you walk along in the sunshine
through the crystal gleaming dew,
It thrills your heart to hear

the bluebirds sing their love to you.
From the apple and the cherry tree,
their joy seems to know no end.
They sing, "If you will let us, we will be your friend."

After the long, cold winter,
God wanted you to know,
That weeds and thorns don't matter,
'cause it's love that really grows.
It's love and joy together
that make me long for spring;
So look beyond the thistle
with its bitter, hurtful sting,
To the promise He has given
of the joy and love of spring.

We do have bad thunderstorms and the occasional destructive tornado in Minnesota. One year we had an early spring storm. The sky grew dark, the wind blew, and the rain poured down. The center of the storm hovered over my parents' suburb. I anxiously listened to the weather report, helpless. I lived about twenty minutes from their house.

Remember, "I'll Praise You in This Storm"? Some storms are worthy of praise, and while it did not seem like it at the time, this storm turned out to be a blessing.

Finally, after the storm subsided, I was able to reach my parents only to find out they had no electricity during the entire storm.

"We couldn't find a flashlight," my mother reported. "But I did find a candle and matches." Why didn't I think of that scenario and make sure they had a flashlight handy?

My husband and I told them to stay there until we could come, which was not to be that night. No travel was allowed in their suburb.

The next day, after the power lines were lifted out of their driveway, my husband and I collected my mother and the food out of the freezer and brought her to our house.

The neighborhood was a mess, with trees and powerlines down everywhere. Dad steadfastly refused to leave so he could protect the house. Whatever, he was wearing me down.

Everyone else in their neighborhood had power back within three days. What about their house? The electricity continued to be out, despite calls to the electric company.

Finally, after a week, a representative came to the house and discovered that the junction box outside in their backyard was old and in bad shape. The storm, fortunately, had totally blown out the box—otherwise, a fire could have started. The electrical box was replaced.

This was also when we discovered the rotting window casings outside.

Maybe, just maybe, that storm turned my father's will a bit. God's hand is in the storm and the calm, and this storm resulted in a visit from a man named Gary.

I believe Gary was sent to us right from the Lord above. Gary, along with his wife, run their own real estate business out of Ramsey, Minnesota. Gary had previously sold a house for Sister 1.

Together with my sisters, we decided to address this issue head on and invited Gary over to give our parents an estimate on the house.

My youngest sister and I joined Gary as he spoke with my parents. Gary is a godly man, who cares more about helping people than making money. We briefed him on the situation and let him do the talking. Gary spoke right to my father, explained the options, and talked about how much money the house could sell for in this neighborhood. At the end of the evening, the miracle happened, and my dad and mother signed the papers to allow Gary to list the house "as is."

Four days after the house went on the market, I received a call from Gary. He had an offer on the house. I was literally shaking as I headed over to my parents' home. It was a good offer from a single woman looking for a home to fix up. They signed the purchase agreement. Not that Dad was happy about this event; he was only doing it for Mom's safety.

Preparing to Move

The whole family swung into high gear. We had a house to sell full of fifty years of stuff! Having lived through the Depression era, my mother did not believe in throwing out things she might need someday. Plus, she still had furniture, pictures, and margarine containers from when her parents passed away. (You never know when a twelve-inch stack of margarine containers might come in handy.)

Where to start?

Fortunately, due to my mother's organizational skills in her younger days, her pictures were in albums, extra canned goods were lined up neatly on the pantry shelves, and the boxes and bags—and margarine containers—were neatly sorted.

I wondered why she had so many cans of brown beans on the pantry shelf downstairs. She had forgotten about them, as she was not going downstairs very often. "We like beans, they can be a whole meal!" mom explained. Unfortunately most of the beans were expired, so we slipped them into the trash.

My brother-in-law hauled away trailer after trailer full of stuff to the junkyard. My mother never, ever threw out foam packing material; there were boxes of it in the basement in case a radio or TV had to be returned.

Sister 4, who packed up almost the whole basement herself, said, "I could handle boxes in boxes and bags in bags. But when I got to the tubes in tubes, I lost it!"

The basement was "appliance" heaven, including an old dead stove used for baking pies at Thanksgiving, two hot water heaters, a water softener, and several washers and dryers. My teenage son grabbed several of his friends, including one big guy from the football team. We rented an "appliance mover" that walks appliances up the stairs. The kids hauled seven dead appliances upstairs. Fortunately, the buyer agreed to keep the giant freezer in the basement.

We became experts at getting rid of stuff. A guy at work was thrilled to take the old stereo cabinet. The Salvation Army would pick up furniture, and they came for the ugly old brown couch, chairs, and side tables.

Later, after they moved, my dad was displeased about losing the brown couch. My aunt gave them one of her couches, but it was smaller, and he couldn't lie all the way down on it. While I felt bad about getting rid of the brown couch, it would not have fit in their new townhome.

While Sister 4 packed and organized the basement, we hired someone to do the cleaning, as none of the sisters cared to encounter the lurking spiders that surely had inhabited the corners for years.

I'm sure it was hard for my parents to see their house dismantled, especially my dad.

However, consider the year we sold the house, 2007. You may recall that the housing bust started in 2008. My parents made enough money from the house to get out of debt and bank money for future expenditures.

Had we waited a year or two, housing prices dropped, and the outcome would likely have been disastrous.

"I will provide," God had promised me.

We three local sisters visited multiple housing options, even before the house was on the market. We visited expensive senior housing complexes with progressive care levels, independent living, and assisted living. We knew money would be an issue. I was grateful we had started to check out housing options before my parents had to move.

They needed to be in a one-level, handicap-accessible home. My mother's main desire was to have her own washer and dryer, (a.k.a. the promise Dad made when he proposed. She took it to heart.)

I knew just the place! A friend of ours was in a complex providing continuous care for its residents. It went from independent apartments to assisted living to a nursing home. Her daughter told us they promised her mom could stay there until the end—they would move her into nursing care if necessary. "We take care of our own" was their motto.

Right before Mom's surgery, we took them to look at the complex. All was going well, until my father went off wandering on his own. He came back red in the face.

"We are not living here!" he announced.

"Why not?"

"The Catholic church is right down the hall!"

My goodness, you would have thought there was a torture chamber down the hall.

It is important to point out the times they had lived through. There was a deep division between the Catholics and Protestants in the fifties and sixties. In my grade school years, the Protestants were sure all the Catholics would go to hell, and the Catholics were sure the Protestants wouldn't be in heaven. Later in life, my father had many Catholic friends, but I believe his dementia aggravated old prejudices.

They did not move into that facility.

The sale of the house coincided with my mother's kidney surgery, which also collided with the need to find just the right living situation. Mom was unable to accompany us on more housing visits.

We were becoming frustrated when a friend told me about a housing complex nearby. They had a series of one-level villas, along with a senior living apartment and nursing home on the premises. Dad agreed and signed the lease agreement for a three-bedroom, one-level villa. It had reduced "tax-credit" pricing, which meant their rent would be $200 less than similar units. There was a washer and dryer in the unit, and it had garage. It was perfect, God's provision. I also marvel about the friends and acquaintances who were gracious and helpful just when we needed it most during this journey.

Ironically, the housing complex was owned by Mary T, an entrepreneur who provided housing for seniors, the disabled, and other people needing housing. She was also a devoted Catholic. (I'm not sure my father ever realized Mary T was Catholic, and I was not about to tell him!)

At My Wits End

Mom was home from the hospital and the rehabilitation facility by the day of the move. It was a hot July day. I woke up in the morning and burst into tears. My husband, bless his heart, is sometimes oblivious. He looked at Sister 2, the guardian angel sister who came to town to help, and said, "What's wrong with her?!"

My sister answered emphatically, "She's exhausted!"

I was, but we survived the day and the move. My uncle in Brainerd had a moving company, and he and my aunt brought their big truck. They saved the day! Another aunt came to keep my mom company while we carried out boxes and sweated.

One very important step we took was to remove dad's guns from his home. Dad was a hunter in younger days, and he owned a shotgun, rifle, and a pistol. The old dad was extremely cautious with guns, but this dad with dementia might not have understood the consequences of what a gun could do. The men in the family were the ones who were insistent we move the guns.

The house was supposed to close the next Monday. Gary called. "Nance, I have some bad news. The buyer's loan didn't go through. They initially approved it, but now they say she hasn't been in her job long enough. We're not closing Monday."

Oh, great, I thought. Now what?

The house did not close the next Monday. I had been counting on the house money to pay their down payment and rent in the villa, and we were $1,000 short. My husband and I had $500 in savings we could lend them, but no one else could come up with the additional funds. (Yes, we were rather broke in those years.)

What to do?

My parents were able to move into the villa since I thought the money would come in a week. But there were further delays, and we did not know if the house deal would fall apart all together.

I made a few calls and landed on the county VA office. Did they have anything for veterans in a crisis? The helpful gentleman on the phone said he would check and get back to me.

Long story short, the Disabled American Veterans (DAV) lent my parents $1,000, just what they needed until the house closed. The representative drove to meet Dad and personally handed him the check. Dad felt good about this; he was able to tap into his Navy service history, and he knew the money would be paid back when the house closed.

Finally, the closing was scheduled for three weeks later. The lady buying the house had to reapply for a mortgage, and she was then approved. My parents had already signed off on the paperwork, so I just needed to go to the closing office. I jumped in my car on another scorching hot July day.

Guess what song came on the radio— "Praise You In This Storm."

The house closed, and we needed to decide what to do with the mortgage check, and the sooner the better.

I talked to our financial advisor, and he advised we put the money into a bank with part of it in short-term money market accounts.

Together the three of us—Mom, Dad, and I, marched off to the local bank.

The check would take some time to clear since it was from out of state. Marvelous.

We agreed to divide the funds into various accounts. $10,000 was put into one of the bank's money market accounts.

That day the bank deposited my parents' mortgage check. However, the bank made a bad mistake: they immediately tried to transfer $10,000 into the money market account, forgetting the mortgage check was not yet cleared. The $10,000 check bounced to high heaven!

We had written several checks in the previous week, including the rent check, an insurance check, and checks for groceries and a few other purchases.

Bouncing checks everywhere! The trouble was, I didn't know which checks would bounce.

I was at my wits' end. The house closing had been delayed, we had just moved my parents, and it was a hot, hot summer. I do not do well in the heat and humidity.

I went to the bank, and they gave me a letter and said they would cover all the costs.

About seven checks bounced. I had to watch the account for any other bouncing checks. I spent every lunch period at work for the next week on the phone explaining why my parents' checks had bounced. Frustrated, I went back to the bank to further discuss the situation. The branch manager begged me not to tell "anyone else" about the mistake. Fortunately for that person, I was too exhausted to pursue repercussions.

Seriously, it's a surprise I didn't lose my mind right then and there. Fortunately, my sisters, who are all better at arranging and decorating than me, were available to get my parents settled in their new home.

Why couldn't the path have been smooth? Perhaps it was another test of faith. The greatest lessons in life are learned through difficulties.

Changes

My parent's new home was in a nice area, with trees and flowers nearby, as described in this poem:

Come take a walk with me today,
And we'll share many a thing.
Flowers growing near the streams,
And maybe hear the bluebirds sing.

We'll walk 'neath great and lofty trees,
Towering to the skies.
And if we really listen,
We can hear the whip-poor-will cries.

Early in the morning we will see the sparkling dew,
But the glory of the sunset is a special treat for you.
We will hear the night birds calling in the fading of the light,
As we wait and watch together for the coming of the night.

In the quietness and the darkness,
When the stars begin to shine,
We'll know that what we've shared together,
Is a time of joy sublime.

The driving situation was going downhill fast. Our parents' multi-family complex had one entrance into the main road, so only local drivers drove on those streets. Children played kickball and rode their bikes on the roads, which were the roads my parents had to drive through to get out to the main road.

Mom would huddle over the steering wheel, driving slowly and carefully. Because she was short, she always used a padded pillow on the seat.

Dad just drove on through. I shuddered to think of the children playing in his path. Dad's eyesight was failing, and his dementia was worsening. What if a young child ran out to catch a rolling ball, or forgot to stop their bike on time? Dad finally agreed to not drive at night and to stay off the highways as much as possible. But he would forget.

I mentioned that one of his side businesses was mini donut-making. Dad seldom made donuts anymore as he had trouble figuring out how to run the machine. Despite this, there was an event at the office in Minneapolis, about a twenty-minute drive on freeways. Dad just had to go and make his famous mini donuts. It was not scheduled to end until after dark. I warned him this was a bad idea.

Dad, being a stubborn dad—and now a dad with dementia—proceeded anyway. It was dark when he drove home, and he admitted later he could not see very well. On the way home a local police officer stopped him. This time he ticketed Dad and said he could not drive until a formal evaluation took place.

Surely an answer to prayer.

Dad was a patient at a VA clinic, so we made an appointment for the driving evaluation. Other local agencies also provide this type of testing; however, he would not have to pay at the VA. I anxiously waited in the family room, trying to read but unable to concentrate. Would someone finally take Dad off the road? If they did, how would he react?

The therapist came out with Dad, who looked troubled. "I'm sorry," she reported. "Your father did not pass the driver's test. He will not be allowed to drive anymore."

I was relieved, but sad. Another step in taking away his independence. It was a very quiet ride home. Dad did not want to stop for our usual pie outing at Nelson Brothers Restaurant in Clearwater, Minnesota.

The driving saga ended, but it opened a whole new set of problems and opportunities.

When my mother-in-law, who lived in another state, couldn't drive anymore, her son conveniently removed the distributor cap and kept the keys for her car. Whenever we talked to my husband's mom, she told us her son would be over the next day to give her keys back. My brother-in-law did faithfully visit her nearly every day, but it was to check on her and bring her groceries and supplies. Mysteriously, the keys never reappeared.

Dad, still irate about the house sale, became sullen. He said he was "stuck in the brush" in the new villa. We lined up Metro Mobility, a service offered by the local city bus company for seniors or disabled individuals. We scheduled trips for him to the store, church, or wherever he wanted to go. When Metro Mobility was not available or we had family outings, my husband, sisters or and me would drive him wherever he needed to go.

We couldn't bear to move Dad out of the office in Minneapolis after taking him out of his house. He still "worked" on his side businesses, and I continued to pay the rent and phone bill for his office. I agreed to drive Dad back and forth to work several days a week. Was it a "coincidence" that my office was only a couple of miles away from Dad's office? Or was it another way God provided for my parents' needs?

Looking back, those times in the car with Dad were precious. It was the closest Dad and I ever "danced" in harmony.

A local church handed out free coffee once a week in the winter, so we made it a habit to drive through for the hot cup. Dad and I loved our coffee!

My dad was an amazing storyteller. As we drove to work, he told me family stories, like the one about great-grandma and the wolves. I wasn't sure if this story was true or part of his dementia-related imagination, until I found a fuller version of the story in a letter Dad wrote to his niece in 1984.

My Great Grandma ("GG") and Grandpa, first generation immigrants from Norway, lived in Grygla, Minnesota. Great Grandpa went to Minneapolis to work, leaving GG to tend the family on a little hard rock, tamarack, swampy farm. They had a few cattle and chickens, and Great Grandma tended a big garden for food. Animals roamed the nearby woods, including huge timber wolves.

One night when GG went to get the cows in, the wolves started circling the cows and her, moving closer and closer. I'm sure GG's heart pounded while she looked desperately for an escape route. The cattle went wild and started running for the barn. GG grabbed a heifer by the tail and sailed along over the landscape.

GG made it to safety, but otherwise she might have been like Little Red Riding Hood, eaten by a wolf.

"The Office"

Dad said he had always wanted to be a minister, which was new information to me. He decided to start a Bible study called "Tuesday Church" in his office. (This church had to be on Tuesday, because, as he mentioned, Sunday was taken.) He had me make up "Tuesday Church" flyers, and he handed them out to the other office residents and people he met on the street. He had a few people attend "Tuesday Church" where he read the Bible and shared the Gospel of Jesus.

The office building was also his social setting. Dad headed upstairs to the coffee shop for his daily donut and had soup for lunch. Northeast Minneapolis is an artistic community, and this office building rented to several artists. Dad knew everyone; he never met someone who did not become a friend.

I remember the day Dad called me in a panic. Someone was looking for a china pot he was supposed to repair, and he couldn't find it. I think he had had it for months because he hadn't done any repair jobs for some time.

I called the lady at the nonprofit who was looking for the teapot. It was an expensive item, valued in the hundreds of dollars, and they needed it that weekend for an auction. He was supposed to have returned it long ago. I consulted with Sister 1, who helped him in the office from time to time. She told me where to look, but the pot was lost.

Finally, Dad said to call "Cary," a down-and-out soul he had rescued by hiring her to work in the office from time to time. Cary said, "Look under his desk, that is where I find his lost items."

Fortunately, I found the box with the lost pot, he was able to make the repair, and it was picked up that day.

My overall anxiety level was rising again.

It eventually became clear that Dad could not afford to keep the office. The rent and phone added up to several hundred dollars a month. He had lost the ability to do almost all his hobbies, glass grinding, donut making, or carving wooden signs. It had been some time since he had been able to get the letters straight in the signs. Hesitatingly, sadly, Dad agreed, and it came to us to get rid of all the stuff that had accumulated. I felt totally overwhelmed.

Sister 1 cheerfully set out to clean out the office with Dad. (You may note that I excel at paperwork but became quite busy when it was time to clean icky, smelly, or spidery places, which completely described his "office.")

It was a ton of work. Sister 1 spent several weekends painstakingly sorting through old paints, pieces of wood, leftover glasses, papers, and a lot of other stuff.

I gave notice to his landlord. She let me know they adored Dad; he always stopped in to say "Hi" and had great stories and jokes. *But* they had given him a good deal on the rent for years; now they could split up the space and charge the market rate.

Such amazing people Dad had in his life.

I found out from the landlord that Dad had been dumping large amounts of garbage from the house into the dumpster, which was costing them money. They had just figured out it was him. Sometimes it is better to not know what has transpired with a loved one.

The final day at the office came. It was sad, something we didn't want to see happen. Dad said goodbye to the coffee shop crew and shook hands with his artist friends.

You see, dementia chips away at life and dignity, piece by piece. It breaks hearts, not only for the person with dementia, but for the loved ones who watch the pieces of life fall apart.

Now he was truly "stuck in the brush."

We had told Dad we would set up an "office" for him in the garage, where he could do his glass grinding and woodworking. He would putz around in the garage, but he missed the social life and was unable to make money at his hobbies. His brain-hand-eye coordination was not connecting like it did for the old Dad.

I had excellent ideas as to what my dad could do with his newfound time at home. He and my mom could go over to the senior apartment building and have lunch with the other seniors.

No, that wouldn't work; they had their own food.

Between the two of them, my parents could be so stubborn!

I took Dad to the drop-in "Adult Day Care" at the nursing home, which was within walking distance. He took one look and said no, this was not for him. Those people there had "that crazy disease" (Alzheimer's, as you may recall).

Dad did make his own path. He ventured over to the nursing home often, not to go to the adult day care (oh, no!) but to meet with nursing home residents. He would bring his big-print Bible and read and pray with the residents. He was known all over the halls.

I registered him for a limited mobility bus he could schedule (with help) so he could go to church, out for lunch, or to Walmart. Walmart was his favorite outing.

One day at work I received a call from my mother. Dad had not come home on the bus as scheduled. I called the bus company; no, he had not gotten on the limited mobility bus. I knew he was going to Walmart, so I called my husband and asked him to run to Walmart to see if Dad was waiting for the bus.

My husband drove to Walmart and looked for my dad. The door greeter reported that an elderly gentleman with a hat had fallen asleep in the chair, but Dad was nowhere to be found.

Where was Dad?

Eventually, my mother called to say Dad had arrived home, a bit winded, but okay. I stopped by after work—Where were you, Dad? My mother rolled her eyes in the background (a common family trait). Dad said his bus didn't come, so he got on the regular county bus. It went around and around; he went by our house a couple of times. Finally, it was the end of the driver's route. The driver couldn't figure out where Dad lived, so he dropped him off at a gas station about three-quarters of a mile from my parents' house.

My dad walked home. Amazingly, he kept his sense of direction for a long time.

I was furious!

I called the bus company. They said, "He needs to be able to manage to get on the bus on his own." I said they should not drop a disabled person off at a random gas station!

Dad did not understand why I was upset—he had managed to get home just fine.

Sigh.

Chapter 8

Resources and Responsibility

We all have our gifts, talents and passions. The Bible talks about the gift of "administration", which is one of my gifts. (I would have preferred to be gifted in singing or art , but God didn't ask me, and He saw fit to give me the gift of administration.) I am also resourceful. When I took the "Strengthfinder" assessment by Tom Rath and the Gallup Poll (now "CliftonStrengths") my greatest strength is "Learner". Administration, resourcefulness, learner, all helpful gifts as I sought to make the best life for my parents in difficult situations. I want to share the ways I was able to use my gifts to assist my family.

Last Will and Testament

I asked my mother, "Where are your wills?"

My organized mother knew exactly where every piece of paper was filed. Out came a faded, handwritten document.

The will was from 1963, before our youngest sister was born. Should my parents die prematurely, it left the three older sisters and their remaining assets to our maternal grandparents. It was a bit outdated since my grandparents had passed away and the *four* of us sisters were adults.

I informed my parents we would be updating their wills. (This was not an option.)

Before going to the attorney, I consulted with my sisters as to who should be the executor and alternate. They all agreed I should be in charge and Sister 4 should be second. The "assets" would be split between the four of us (which was ultimately a non-issue, as there were no assets left).

I found an attorney recommended by the American Association of Retired Persons (AARP), and off I went with my parents to set their affairs in order.

The attorney helped us complete wills, power of attorney documents, and medical power of attorney/living will/advance directives.

To sign legal documents, you must be "of sound mind." I hoped the attorney would not deem Dad unfit. He was able to sign the paperwork and answer questions.

The attorney sent the advanced care directive home for us to complete. My mother assured us she wanted no extra measures; when it was her time to go, she wished to pass on without any artificial means of resuscitation. This is called DNR - Do Not Resuscitate. (In spite of having this document, at every hospital visit they would ask again if her desire was DNR.)

My father was another story. He did (sort of) agree that there should be no extra measures to keep him alive. When it came to the specific questions, he became confused.

"Dad, do you want any extra measures to prolong your life?"

"No."

Dad could not make specific decisions regarding care should he become incompetent.

"Do you want a feeding tube?"

"I don't know."

"How about hydration, like an IV?"

"A what?"

"Do you want medications?"

"Don't ask me all that."

Finally, I said, "Dad, let's just put down it's up to your caregivers."

"Yes. Okay."

My sisters were happy to have me as primary in all those areas. I was the "administrative" sister, after all. This was not like winning a popularity contest. It is a lot of work and decision-making. I was careful to run all major decisions by my sisters and always offered to let them review the financial paperwork. Sister 4 was secondary on all documents.

Acting on Dad's Behalf

How hard is it to act on behalf of a person? Below are situations I ran into with my dad shortly after his dementia diagnosis.

Dad wanted a couple of stations added to his cable TV roundup. I stopped at the house and told him I would call the cable company, and they might need to talk to him to confirm that I could change his account. He agreed.

"Hello, I'd like to make some changes to my dad's cable TV account."

"Is this Lee Eggerud?"

"No, this is his daughter."

"I can only speak to Lee because the account is in his name."

"Okay, I will put him on, and he will let you know it's okay to talk to me."

I put Dad on the phone.

"Yes, Lee, is it okay if your daughter speaks for you on your cable TV plan?"

Dad: "No, don't listen to her! Don't do anything she says!"

Sigh. Eye roll. From there on, we rehearsed in advance what we would say on the phone.

My dad insisted on getting another opinion on his glaucoma, so his eye doctor sent him to the local university physicians. I thought, what could go wrong with this visit? I assumed the original eye doctor had forwarded the medical records.

I dropped him off, went back to work, and picked him up an hour later.

Dad said, "That doctor says there's something wrong with me. Not just my eyes." A week later a letter arrived. Here is part of it:

"Thank you for asking me to see Lee in Neuro-ophthalmic consultation. Unfortunately, he is a very, very poor historian [it went on to state the confusion on Dad's part and listed pictures of people he couldn't recognize.] However . . . he is able to recognize a picture of Superman."

It went on to say he should have an MRI to obtain a diagnosis.

Clearly, I should have been at the doctor appointment. To set the record straight, I called the physician's office at the university. This was shortly after the HIPAA privacy regulations went into place.

I spoke to someone in the office and told him I had information about Lee.

"I can't tell you anything," the young man who answered the phone said to me.

"That's okay," I said. "I can tell you information."

"I don't think so," he insisted.

"Yes, I can, and here is the situation. He has dementia, it has been diagnosed. . . ."

(I had written about privacy regulations in graduate school, so I had a good idea of what was allowed.)

Support

My mother and I attended a support group for family members of dementia patients. While my mother didn't talk much, I believe we both were helped by hearing other people's stories.

When I told the head of our department, an attorney, about my dad, he got tears in his eyes and told me his grandmother had Alzheimer's. My workplace/employer was understanding and supportive during the caretaking years. I was conscientious, working late the next day when I missed my regular work hours. (I am my father's daughter after all.)

Veterans Association (VA)

The VA helped in many ways. We took him to a VA medical clinic in St. Cloud, Minnesota. I have nothing but praise for their care. He was able to receive medications at no charge, a free blood pressure machine, and the attention of multiple caregivers at each visit. Every single person was helpful and respectful to my dad.

I attended several dementia conferences. It was there I heard about "Aid and Attendance," a pension offered by the VA for homebound vets sixty-five and over. I found it by searching "Aid and Attendance" on the Americanverteransaid website.

My father qualified to the various requirements, and I set about filling out the paperwork. I discovered how archaic the federal VA system was in 2007. Change of address forms were sent multiple times. I filled out the correct form giving me permission to speak for him, yet every time I spoke with a representative, they had to dig through electronic paperwork to find the correct form. I imagine the forms were scanned in without being categorized.

The Veterans' Service Organization (or VSO), a private non-government group, was very helpful. Several times they told me the exact wording to put on the government forms to get through the system. I later found out they would have filled out the paperwork, but I didn't mind taking care of it myself. The VSO is another great resource.

Months later Dad was finally approved. He received back pay and a healthy monthly allotment supplementing my parents' Social Security and house savings.

I hope the VA system has improved their paperwork and computer systems. The federal employees were always helpful; however, I could sense their frustration. Our veterans struggle enough; let's not let paperwork bring them down.

Medical Assistance

I still had concerns about money and looked for ways to get their medical premiums paid.

While on Medicare, nearly $100 a month for Medicare premiums came out of their Social Security checks. In addition, they had to pay between $150 and $200 a month for their supplemental medical plans.

I filled out the county paperwork for Medical Assistance (also called "Medicaid"). To apply, I needed all sorts of records, such as birth certificates, military records, marriage and divorce papers, bank records, home sale reports, car titles, and much, much more. Fortunately my mom had nearly everything I one folder.

My parents did not qualify for Medical Assistance as they had too many assets. (Too many assets being greater than $3,000 at that time.) However, several years later when I finally completed all this paperwork for my dad to obtain Medical Assistance, I had all the information ready.

Tracking Expenses

I continued to carefully watch their income and expenses, making spreadsheets and carefully tracking their finances. My mother was a great partner in this endeavor. Until almost the end of her life, she was careful with money, a good accountant, and kept track of their important papers.

I used a simple Excel spreadsheet and kept their receipts and other important documents where I could easily find them if needed.

My mom taught me the importance of keeping track of important documents in an organized manner. She also made certain at least one other family member could find paperwork when needed.

Chapter 9

Life Goes On

Now that Dad wasn't driving, it became harder to get him to Dr. S. in Minneapolis. I had a lot of respect for Dr. S, but not his clinic. The problem was twofold:

- He was primarily on faculty at a local university; he only saw patients a couple times a month. It was difficult to get appointments.
- Dr. S practiced at a run-down clinic in an old part of town. Staff at his clinic were hard to reach, they had no phone messaging system. I would call, and often the phone would ring and ring with no answer. (I'm sure when my father was making his own appointments, he just stopped in to chat with the scheduling staff.)

So when Dad needed medical care, I decided to schedule him to see a doctor at my suburban clinic.

The Prostate Medication Fiasco

Prostate trouble . . . not something a daughter wants to think about with her father. However, when you go to medical appointments with a loved one, you learn about various conditions. Dad had started taking a drug to shrink his prostate, which addresses urination problems. Dad said his prostate was getting worse.

When I requested an appointment at my clinic with a physician treating seniors, they scheduled Dad with a family practice physician. However, when we saw the doctor, he informed us he primarily saw pediatric patients and teens—why were we seeing him? (I wondered also.) At my father's report of his urination difficulties, this doctor increased my dad's dose of prostate medication by a large amount.

Long story short, the prescription was too high of a dose.

The next day, I dropped by dad off at his office in Minneapolis and headed to my own work. Dad proceeded to get quite dizzy (more dizzy than normal) and fell and cut his head open. Ever resourceful and independent, he took a bus to a familiar clinic, had the cut cleaned up, and returned to his office without alerting anyone in the family. At the end of the day when I picked him up, I wondered why his head was bandaged up. With some difficulty, he told me the bus story.

I later learned this prostate medication should only be increased in small increments. Why the doctor had prescribed a high dose, I do not know, perhaps because he did not regularly treat seniors. Dad never saw him again, and I didn't pursue the topic. However, my father, forgetful though he was, did not forget that incident! He told it over and over. I even received a call from my aunt "informing" me of this situation. (I didn't know if it would be better to tell her I knew about the situation, or to just keep quiet, so I kept quiet. This is a good example of how I danced around the real story!)

Had I only known how hard it would be to find a gerontologist we would not have changed doctors. It is so important for a person to trust their medical team—how much more when you cannot think straight, and your mind is telling you not to trust people you do not know. We would have stuck with Dr. S.

Until Dad entered a nursing facility, we could not settle on a family physician, although he did get excellent care from the VA. I'm sure he resented me taking him away from Dr. S.

Much later we found an excellent medical team in his long-term care facility specializing in dementia. Or more accurately, they found us.

Steady State

The next year was, for the most part, steady state for our parents. While Dad wasn't particularly happy about his new situation, he made his way around via the mobility bus, found old friends, and made new ones. He was generally a happy guy who loved to tell stories and jokes. The jokes by this time were repetitive because he couldn't remember a lot of them, but we would just smile and chuckle right along with him. It was good to have humor.

He especially liked old family anecdotes. I reminded him about the first time I mentioned "I met someone," my future husband. My dad's first question was "Does he have a job?" I assured him, yes, he has a job. My dad would get a little smile and throaty chuckle when we'd bring up this type of story. (Yes, I married someone like my workaholic dad—my husband, now retired, loved nothing better than going to work and would not call in sick unless he absolutely could not get out of bed.)

My mother seemed to recover well from her kidney surgery. They said it was Stage 2 and confined to the surgically removed kidney. No more treatment was required, and the doctor did not see a need for mom to consult an oncologist.

I had a work colleague, "Dr. M," who was a physician at the University of Minnesota. One of her specialties was Renal Cell Carcinoma, the type of cancer that took my mother's kidney. Dr. M was supportive throughout this process.

The kidney protocol recommended my mother have periodic scans to make certain the cancer hadn't spread. She had one X-ray the first year, but no MRI-type scans were ordered by her family practice physician.

A year and a half went by. My mother took care of my dad and herself mentally, sorting their medications and making easy lunches and dinners. My dad took care of her physically, making their toast in the morning when mom was sleepy and doing simple household tasks. We hired a former neighbor to clean house. My mother liked her; she was not only a house cleaner, but a pleasant companion for my mother.

Fire!

And then there was the fire. (My dad's second fire—you may recall the first one when he and his sister burned down the barn.)

I stopped by my parents' house one day on the way home from work.

My mother stated, "I can't get the window closed all the way after the fire."

"What fire?"

Her eyes got big and she clasped her hand over her mouth. "I wasn't supposed to tell you about the fire!"

The secret was out, so I insisted she tell me. Dad had microwaved a muffin too long, and it caught on fire. My mother pushed the button on her emergency call system necklace, calling for emergency help. The fire department came screeching to the villa.

There was smoke, but no other damage. The firemen opened all the windows to let out the smoke. Later my mother managed to close the windows, other than the one that got stuck in the spare bedroom.

We unstuck the window and closed it. I just shook my head.

Fear may be your companion when a relative has dementia. Will they get hurt, will they walk in front of a car, will they burn the house down?

Or you can just be thankful that when something happens, it turns out okay.

Here is another example of what can happen with dementia—and without it! While my dad was still driving, my parents went to a concert in downtown Minneapolis. He left the car running in the parking garage the whole time they were at the concert. Luckily, it didn't run out of gas.

Wouldn't you know it? A couple of months later, my husband and I went out to dinner, and guess who left the car running the whole time we were eating in the restaurant? ME!

We all have accidents; we all do dumb things. I learned when I was quick to judge my dad for his lapses, I was also just human, and sometimes made the same mistakes.

Breath of Life

Sometime later I received a call at work. "I'm having a lot of trouble breathing," my mother gasped.

"Push the button on your necklace!" I told her.

The ambulance brought her to the local hospital. Her lung had collapsed, seemingly for no reason. As I was driving to the hospital, "Praise You In This Storm," by Casting Crowns came on the radio.

I heard God whisper to me in the storm, *"She will die from lung collapse."*

Really? Did God speak to me again? (You may recall, I heard the voice of God when He told me He would take care of their finances)

Well, mom did not die, not yet anyway. They fixed up her lung and sent her home. Was it my imagination? The voice stuck in my head.

Mom was enthralled with Dr. B. I had several conversations with Dr. B about my mother's health through those final years.

I researched renal cell carcinoma and learned that when it metastasized, the first place it goes is to the lungs. The oncologist had said she should have MRIs periodically to see if the cancer had spread.

I called Dr. B and asked, "Could this possibly be the cancer spreading to her lungs?" He replied, "That's a good question, but no, we don't see any indication of cancer from the X-rays." I wondered why he was doing X-rays and not the MRI but did not ask. I preferred to believe her cancer had been contained as it was easier to be in denial.

I had a random conversation with a top oncologist on an airplane regarding my mother's cancer. He highly recommended we take her to an oncologist immediately. We didn't. She was over eighty years old and did fine—after her lung was re-inflated.

Human beings have an amazing ability to adapt and cope with change. Mother returned home from the hospital, and our parents continued to adjust to their changing status. It was steady state with a slight continuous downward slope.

The voice telling me Mom would die from the lung collapse stayed in back of my mind, but I thought it was my imagination.

Chapter 10

Not the Spring We Expected

Do you feel the shadows falling,
Like a blanket falling down?
Great flakes of snow, of darkness,
As a goose would lose its down—
This is loneliness and sorrow.

This is sadness coming down
When love and light come back
Upon the scene of life
And we're free from lonely suffering.

Why is lonely like a darkness
That suddenly sweeps across your face,

And it seems like even God
Has taken away from you His grace?

March in Minnesota is usually still winter. April is one of those in-between-months. It might snow or rain. Flowers poke out of the earth and trees begin to bud. It is a season of hope.

This spring was not what we expected. After a year of relative calm, in late March 2009 I received a call at work from my brother-in-law. My dad had tried to call me, then he tried my youngest sister, and finally reached her husband. My brother-in-law reported, "Your mother can't breathe, and your dad doesn't know what to do!"

I called my dad, who was in a panic and could barely articulate the words about my mom. I said, "Dad – push the button on Mom's necklace!"

"The what?"

"The button on her necklace, Dad!"

"Okay." A minute of silence, then he returned to the phone. "I pushed it and they said they will send an ambulance."

"Good job, Dad!" I said in relief.

I also called the helpful sisters across the street from my parents, who promptly came over to wait with them for the ambulance. The ambulance driver came, I talked to him on the phone and said I would meet my mom at the local hospital. I left work and met her in the emergency room where she was pale and being assessed by the doctors. I am not very good in a medical crisis, and I was getting worn out, so I called my oldest sister, who quickly came. I started to cry and told her I couldn't cope. Sister 1 told me to just go home and she would wait with our mother. Bless her loving, caretaking heart.

A Broken Heart

They admitted mom to the hospital to assess her status and to inflate her lungs, which had both collapsed.

This time was very stressful for all of us. Dad became confused again; sometimes he talked like his wife was his mother, or he couldn't remember when we were going to the hospital.

Dad had a congenital heart defect, and when he was stressed, his heart would beat fast. (It could have been repaired when he was in his fifties, but he decided he could control it—he just needed to lie down and his heart would go back to normal.) One night we were leaving the hospital and he clutched his chest.

"I have to lie down!"

"Let's just go to the emergency room, Dad."

"No! I just have to lie down until my heart slows down."

He lay down in the back of my car, hands crossed over his heart, and waited for his heartbeat to subside. When his heart returned to normal, we headed home.

Coming Home

Thank goodness for multiple sisters—we could share the duties of visiting our mother in the hospital and taking care of Dad. Sister 2 came from out East and spent many nights sleeping in the hospital next to our mother. As time progressed, we learned that both lungs had collapsed, and the cancer had spread to her lungs. At first, they thought she had lung cancer, but then identified kidney cancer cells. It was terminal.

Sister 2 was there (thank goodness) when they talked to Mom about receiving palliative care and ultimately about accepting hospice care. After twenty days in the hospital, Mom moved home, along with oxygen, two long tubes hanging off her chest to keep her lungs inflated, pain pills, and a hospice plan. This was on a Monday.

(I later discovered that Medicare will only cover twenty-one days of hospital care. After nearly three weeks of what felt like nothing happening, amazingly on the twentieth day, they said she could go home.)

After Mom came home, Dad became very ill, with throwing up and diarrhea. I called the clinic, and they said he could have caught C. diff (Clostridium difficile, a contagious disease, at times spread in hospitals.)

I took him into the clinic, and as he was talking to the doctor, I burst into tears. "I'm sorry, my mother is home dying."

The doctor was kind and understanding, even though I wasn't the patient. I literally had very little emotional reserve left.

The culture showed he did not have C. diff. If it wasn't C. diff, was it still contagious or just stress?

I learned it was contagious.

What was to be the night before Mom died, Sister 2 had us all come to the villa for a meeting. How should we proceed to care for Mom? The physician said she could live three or four months, but once Sister 2 went home, Dad couldn't take care of her. Amazingly, Mother agreed to go to the local nursing home and perhaps be able to come home during the day.

The next day I stopped at my parents' house on the way to work. My sister reported that Mom had a painful, stressful night; she had had to call the hospice nurse at two a.m. A high dose of morphine was administered in hopes she might snap out of it by the next day.

Little Mother didn't come out of it. As the day progressed, the family gathered around. We cried, we prayed, we held her hand. I tried to read her the 23rd Psalm, but I couldn't get through it without breaking up. Yet it gave me comfort. Here it is in the King James version, which my mother faithfully read daily.

The 23rd Psalm

The Lord is my shepherd; I shall not want.
He maketh me to lie down in green pastures:
he leadeth me beside the still waters.
He restoreth my soul:
he leadeth me in the paths of righteousness for his name's sake.
Yea, though I walk through the valley of the shadow of death,
I will fear no evil: for thou art with me;
thy rod and thy staff they comfort me.
Thou preparest a table before me in the presence of mine enemies:
thou anointest my head with oil;
my cup runneth over.
Surely goodness and mercy shall follow me all the days of my life:
and I will dwell in the house of the Lord forever.

By mid-afternoon we were a little goofy. My niece and sister decided we were to give our comatose mother/grandmother death-bed confessions.

My niece said she had sneakily taken candy out of my mother's dresser drawer when grandma wasn't looking.

I said in seventh grade I secretly put on eye shadow after I left the house and took it off before I got home from school.

My dad walked around in a daze, sometimes sitting next to her, sometimes going out to the garage.

At about 5 p.m. on April 3, 2009, five days after she came home from hospice, Mom slipped into the welcome arms of Jesus.

O friend to take that blessed leap
Beyond this land of eternal sleep
Until that time when we shall keep
Our souls where mortals no more weep
Where the light of God rules night and day
And saints and angels live and play
And we shall hear our Jesus say,
"This is your 'forever' holiday".

(We should have known she was aware she was dying—Mom never would have agreed to go into the nursing home under normal circumstances!)

The still, small voice came back to me. Yes, mom died of the lung collapse, but she entered a better place where there is no sickness or sorrow.

I was lost. I was my mother's confidant, her caretaker, her parent. A magazine had printed a picture of a middle-aged woman holding a baby, except the baby was an elderly parent. That is how I felt about my mother.

I was sick, thanks to Dad for passing on the stomach ailment to me.

I was exhausted.

My nephew and his wife came and stayed with us before the funeral. My nephew was at seminary in Missouri and his wife was working to support them both. His sweet wife took over the funeral logistics I would have done if I had not been sick. She worked with our church on the brochures and the music (she was a music/worship major in college). My nephew offered us comfort and ran errands. Again, the Lord provided just what was needed.

Mom's visitation and funeral passed in a blur. Sitting near the casket the night before the funeral, I greeted friends—sick, tired, and hoping I wasn't contagious.

At Mom's request, a good minster friend officiated her funeral, and each of the grandchildren participated. My mother's greatest joy in life was her grandchildren; she adored them, and they adored her.

I mostly tried not to cry but was not successful. It was a memorable service; we have a tape of it, but I haven't listened to it since that day.

I had reached the end of my proverbial rope.

After the funeral I announced to my sisters, "I'm done taking care of people. You three take care of Dad.

I QUIT."

Chapter 11

Onions and Tulips

Love is like a garden,
There are so many different things
Some that make you laugh and cry
And some that make you sing.
Now tulips surely are a sight
Pleasant to the eye,
And onions seem to have the job
Of making people cry.

But who can guess, or even know,
What love is all about?
Sometimes makes you quiet,
And sometimes makes you shout.
How can the very same love,

Both make me laugh and cry?
All I know is wells spring up,
And never do run dry.
Sometimes laughter, sometimes tears,
And often joy will flow.

I grieved for my mother. Grief was my master and I was merely its servant. Grief decided I would hear a song and cry in my car. Grief said, "Be flooded with sadness" at the local theater after her death, because the last time I'd been there was with my mom. I cried when I first wrote this story in my blog, and she had been gone nine years at that time. While I was crying for my mom, I cried about missing my grandparents, missing the good times when we were young and a youth that had flown away.

I cried even more than I cry when I peel an onion.

Did you figure out that my proclamation that I quit did not last very long? I lived the nearest to Dad; we had to bring him meals, sort and administer his medication, and help him adapt to living alone. I could not desert my father. We would fight this battle together.

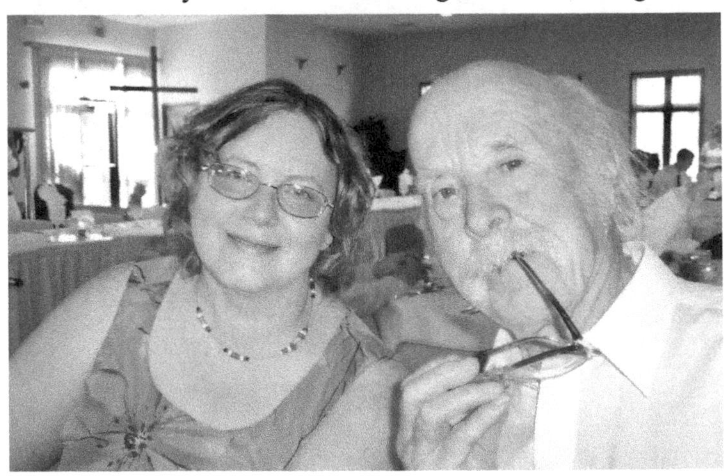

Dad and Me

The Family "Out West"

I had long wanted to take Dad to Seattle to visit family, so this seemed like a good time. We bought tickets with the memorial money from Mom's funeral. I was thrilled when my dad's youngest sister was able to go with us. She's a hoot! About six weeks after my Mother's death, Dad, my aunt, and I boarded an airplane. I was so glad she was along; she knew how to maneuver my Dad around the airport without upsetting him.

My dad had his own room in the hotel, and Auntie and I shared a room. One night, Auntie and I decided we needed a girl's getaway. We figured Dad must be tired—he was eighty-plus years old, and we had been out visiting all day. We said goodnight to him at his door, and Auntie and I snuck off across the street for a glass of wine and "girl talk."

The next day my dad said, "I think your aunt snuck out of the hotel last night!" My eyes got big. "Really Dad—how do you know?"

"I went out to look for a newspaper and saw her leaving!"

"Hmmm . . . ," I said.

The next night the two of us giggled like two schoolgirls and snuck out again. Here we were, two women in our fifties and sixties, ditching our dad/big brother for an outing!

We spent time with my aunt and uncles and their families. We visited my dad's youngest brother in the nursing home. He had Alzheimer's and cancer; his caretaking took a toll on his daughter. He died in 2018, too young. Another life stolen by dementia *and* cancer, two evils that exist in this world.

It is such a blessing we went to Seattle when my dad still knew everyone and was able to travel and visit. Since then, Dad and each of these uncles and aunts have passed away. I had such a great time with Dad and my aunt, but it made her premature death at age sixty-nine several years later all the sadder.

We also visited with various cousins. One of my older cousins and his wife hosted us for a nice dinner. Now I hear from his wife that he is in the beginning stages of Alzheimer's. Will it ever end?

Dad did quite well on the trip, overall. It was a whirlwind, but he loved seeing everyone. We both came back renewed and closer than ever.

Return to Reality

Then, once again, reality struck.

The new reality set in when we got home from Seattle. Dad remained unhappy about moving out of the house and was cross that I controlled his money. In my head I understood this was dementia, but in my heart it hurt.

We were still dancing around the dementia, but it was getting easier and easier to misstep. When I look back at this picture, his hands are in an odd position. Lewy already had his grip on Dad's body.

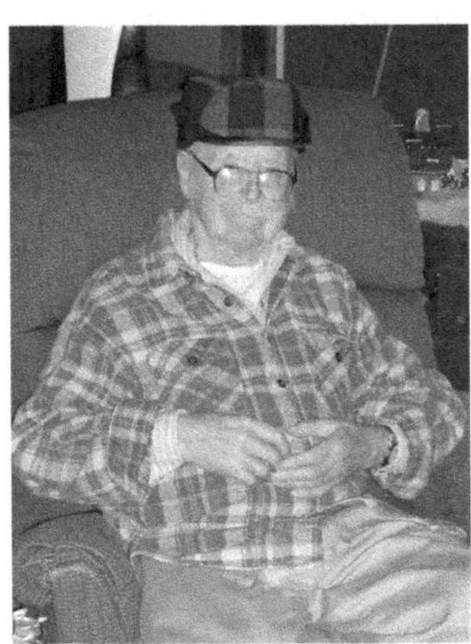

Lewy Hands

The sisters realized he would need to move to a place where he would get more care. He was angry and confused—now he loved his villa "in the brush."

Dad said, "When your mother was alive, we didn't need help with medications."

On another day he said, "When your mother was alive, we could make our own food." He could be obstinate and stubborn.

Love of Horses

To appreciate the next story, let us look back at his growing-up years, where horses were a part of their lives.

When Dad's family lived on the farm, they had a pair of horses named Barney and Mae. Barnie and Mae would be hooked up to a sleigh to haul milk to the milk truck two miles away. In the winter when Grandpa's car wouldn't start, they would hook up the horses to Grandpa's car. With Grandpa at the controls, the kids would run down the road pushing the car while the horses pulled, hoping the car would start.

When it snowed significantly (which if often does in Minnesota) they would hook it up to Barney and Mae up to the old wooden plow to clear the driveway.

Dad said, "I felt so sorry for those horses, breathing in that cold air, slipping and sliding."

Then poor old Mae got sleeping sickness, which was an epidemic. The horse went down and couldn't get up. Dad helped his mom treat the horse. Grandma would hold Mae's head while Dad poured water in her mouth with an extra-large beer bottle. But the poor old horse died, and Dad and his brother had to dig the horse's grave. Maybe this is where my Dad got a soft spot in his heart for horses.

I shared my dad's love of horses. Several of my aunts and uncles had horses, and when we visited them as kids, I'd ride horses with my cousins. I still love to jump on a horse and ride when the opportunity presents itself.

Towards the end of Dad's stay at the Plaza where he lived for a year and a half, he took me to his bookshelf and gave me a pair of horse bookends. They were made of an opaque material. Dad knew I liked horses, and he knew reading was a passion of mine. I'd like to think the horse bookends were something of a conciliatory gift, as we had a number of disagreements I those days. The horse bookends sit on my bookshelf to this day, and I am very fond of the pair.

One day about a year ago, I dropped one of the horse bookends. It cracked and the head fell off—I was horrified. I got to work and glued the head back on, putting the slivers into place. As I was setting it back on the shelf, I noticed a glued crack on the other horse's head. My dad must have glued that bookend together. Strangely, I felt a connection with my dad at that moment—two repaired horse heads, one by each of us.

Back to the housing visits, we sisters trekked around to see various assisted living housing facilities. Dad came with us on one visit; he did not like it because the tour guide talked to us, not him. He may have had brain malfunction, but our dad was still in charge!

We visited several more places including "the Plaza," located in the town where I lived. He asked if he could bring his *horse*, and the tour guide enthusiastically said, "Yes, of course you can!" She was smart, talking directly to Dad, and knew not to disagree with him.

Was he thinking he was back on the farm with Barney and Mae?

She told Dad he could have meals with the other residents. "I don't need meals; I get free food!"

"Dad, how do you get free food?"

"From you girls, of course," and the sheepish smile and throaty chuckle shone through.

I just rolled my eyes and shook my head—behind his back!

We signed him up for a one-bedroom apartment at the Plaza, which was an independent living facility where he had his own apartment, but we could buy-up services such as extra nursing care, house cleaning, additional meals or other services. They had activities for the residences and treated them like family.

Lurking Lewy

I believe Lewy was lurking in the background all this time; we just did not know the name of this insidious disease. We were still rolling with vascular dementia. I don't know if he had dual diseases or the medical community was not familiar enough with Lewy body dementia as that point and did not diagnose from the MRI.

I had never known my dad to be afraid of anything. During times of plenty or times of scarcity, he just plunged on, supporting his family and living his life. But I can imagine how scary this new situation must have been for our strong, independent Dad. Little by little he was losing faculties and independence. We were headed downhill on a roller coaster that would not stop.

Sometimes I look back and wonder if I wasn't empathetic enough, or if I should have tried harder to try to look at life from his vantage point. I know this: As caregivers, we cannot beat ourselves up as to what could have been.

Looking back, life at the Plaza was overall a pleasant interlude. On one hand, I'm glad I did not know what was to come. On the other hand, had we known about Lewy body dementia, could we have done anything to stave off the symptoms?

An Interim Peace

The Plaza was a great place for Dad at this point in his life, and life was relatively peaceful. Dad could get meals, and they had activities and nursing care on site. I had many conversations with the nursing staff—we knew each other by our first names the first week.

There were a few "bugs" to be worked out. The first day they knocked on Dad's door at 8 a.m. and came right into the bedroom to give him his meds! Oh, he was not happy, and with his halting speech, I heard about this intrusion! He said repeatedly he was just going to get himself a little bungalow to live in.

I talked the timing through with the nurses, and they agreed they could wait until later in the morning to give him his meds. They were very nice and caring people, sweet like tulips and roses.

Dad wrote this poem; I am dedicating it to all the paid caregivers.

The pinkest petal on the rose
Is like your love so fair,
It tells me of a gentle heart
And one that's filled with care.

A caring touching fragrance comes
From out that pink bouquet,
That makes your life a flower garden
Of joy from day to day.

The flowers that you grow and give
Are such a joy to share,
One is called "Thoughtfulness,"
Another one is "Care."

Appreciation blossoms
And understanding grows.
"Let me help you" and "I understand"
You see in many rows.

The fragrance from the petals
Of your "Please" and "Thank you" rose,
Are surely among the loveliest
That in your garden grows.

One day the Plaza had a celebration. The local police department closed the street, and they had snacks, a band, and a street dance. My dad shuffled over to the nurse I will call "Ann," and together they "danced" in the street. It was an amazing sight to behold and a happy day during the storm.

Dad got over his initial annoyance and enjoyed going to the meals where he could talk and laugh with people. Ever the helpful guy, he watched over Mabel, an older lady in the building who used a walker. He would make sure Mabel got back to her apartment after dinner, and even escorted her to a couple of events.

Coincidentally, Lola, one of our old neighbors from childhood, lived in the Plaza. Lola and her husband had raised their family across the street from us; I was friends with her daughters. Lola was a staunch Catholic. Here was the perfect opportunity for Dad to convert her to Protestantism—and for Lola, who was as tough as he was—to convert him to Catholicism!

I'm sure it was a friendly exchange that kept them both on their toes. They would debate and laugh together, and I saw a little twinkle in Lola's eyes when she'd "confront" Dad.

Often, he would meet up with Lola and the other gals to watch baseball on TV.

We had good times. Dad attended our church, and he naturally made friends. We'd go out to eat, and he would joke with the waitresses (even though it was the same jokes we had heard a hundred times). Across the street was a river, and we'd stroll in the park until Dad got too tired.

One day we were walking in our small town and he spotted a beading store. He got very excited—apparently beading had been one of his side hobbies. He said he would be back to buy beads!

When he lived at the Plaza, I would often stop in for a visit. A couple of conversations with Dad come to mind.

Wedding Ring

My dad had not worn his wedding ring for years. When Dad moved into the assisted living facility, he insisted on wearing his wedding ring. "I don't want those widows thinking I'm available!"

I had trouble understanding my father when he was lucid; at this point I didn't even try to figure out the wedding ring decision.

One thing continued to be an annoyance to Dad; he was not happy I controlled his money. (In reality, due to the impaired executive functioning in his brain, he could not manage it himself. But I think he would forget and blame the situation on me.)

I gave him whatever cash he needed, but at times he was certain I hid his wallet. He got to the point where he could not write out checks, which I thought was just as well. (He tried to write checks to various appeals he saw on TV; I was not thrilled with some of his choices.) He'd ask me to write checks, and I did for our local church but held off on some other causes.

And yes, of course I was being judgmental. But I still wouldn't change my position on certain causes.

Dad had trouble remembering our names. One time, when he was with all my sisters and me, we asked him where he wanted to go eat. He pointed to me and said: "Ask the bossy one!"

Of course, my sisters thought it was hilarious and still refer to me as "The Bossy One" from time to time. *Well, someone must take charge!*

I stopped to see Dad at the Plaza one sunny afternoon. He was sitting in his favorite recliner; I curled up on the flowered couch. Mom came up in the conversation. Dad said (in his broken way of talking), "God's been dealing with me. Your mom had a hard time of it. If I ever did anything that hurt her or made it worse, I've prayed God will forgive me."

This meant a lot to me, bringing tears to my eyes. They had their share of difficulties, and hindsight gave him clarity, even through the fog of dementia.

I told this to my sisters after he passed away. Sister 4 said this also meant a lot to her; our dad really did have a tender heart and never meant to do wrong to anyone.

Life gets messy; people are born into sin and only made whole through Jesus.

While there is no marriage among humans in heaven, I like to imagine my parents sitting together on a rock, looking at a flowing stream on a sunny day and talking happily about how well their daughters turned out! (Seriously, I am certain the joy of being with the eternal God far outweighs anything on this earth, children or otherwise.)

Morning has come
And the joy of life
Is resplendent in the air.
It's time to rise
And seize the prize
And cast away your care.
There is One above,
The author of love,
Who knows your every care.
So step into the sunlight
This day is yours to share.

Chapter 12

Lewy, Lewy, Out of Hiding

I recall the Nancy Reagan-era commercials: "This is your brain" (picture of a normal brain). "This is your brain on drugs" (picture of a fried egg). Along that line, a brain with Lewy body dementia is quite different from a normal brain.

> *Juebin Huang, MD, PhD, Memory Impairment and Neurodegenerative Dementia (MIND) Center, University of Mississippi Medical Center, wrote:*
>
> *"In Lewy body dementia and Parkinson's disease dementia, abnormal round deposits of a protein (called Lewy bodies) form in nerve cells. Lewy bodies result in the death of nerve cells. In Lewy body dementia, Lewy bodies form throughout the outer layer of the brain (gray matter, or cerebral cortex). The cerebral cortex, which is the largest*

> *part of the brain, is responsible for thinking, perceiving, and using and understanding."*[5]

Dad became progressively more debilitated as time went on.

His shuffled down the halls at the Plaza.

His speech was increasingly hesitant. It was getting harder and harder for him to put sentences together.

"What day to it?"

"Are I going today?"

"I need store." He didn't take the bus anymore; we would drive him.

Dad told one of my sisters he didn't want to go down to meals anymore because "The other guys have stories. I can't anymore."

Oh, the heartache Lewy was bringing our family.

Lewy cells grow slowly in the brain, killing off the good cells. Lewy is insidious.

Lewy was only going to make all our lives worse soon.

Wedding Joy

Happy day—wedding for my cousin's daughter! After the church nuptials we headed to the reception hall. Dad came along, slowly shuffling, stopping on a bench to rest before we found our table in the reception hall. He was wearing down for certain. But he enjoyed visiting with friends and family.

The cousins played instruments while the kids got up to dance. I convinced Dad to get up and dance with me. Because I didn't have a dance at my own small wedding years before, I had seldom danced with him.

He shuffled to the dance floor with me, held me as I tried not to cry. How did I know tonight would be the last time he would hold me in his arms, or we would be able to dance together?

Maybe this poem is a sign of the ramblings in his mind.

I think that you live
In a bubble somewhere;
I've never been there,
So I do not know where
And when you leave here,
I think you go there.

Where is your bubble,
And what do you do?
Are there people and things there.
Waiting for you?

I wonder and ponder
'Cause I don't really know,
That this is a place
Where others can't go.

This place is a place
Just one of a kind
A secret place
You hide in your mind.

If there are other people there,
Nobody can see
And often I wonder

If one of them is me.

Well, I really shan't worry
'Cause I think I may know;
Search as we may,
We never can go

My body's not there,
It's right here with me
So I'm sure your bubble's
A mind place, you'll see.

So when you get to your bubble,
No one knows where
And you see us, please tell us
How did we get there?

Two weeks later, another cousin had a wedding for her son; a fun, informal outdoor occasion. Dad also came to this one.

We were in a park with a big circular pavilion. Dad was acting strangely, walking back and forth, back and forth, head down, not talking to anyone. He would not sit down and barely ate.

My oldest sister, my husband, and I exchanged looks. We tried walking with him, but he seemed oblivious to us. Family members who had seen him and talked with him just a couple of weeks ago tried to talk to him, but he barely glanced their way.

We took him home early, wondering what was going on. Had something in his brain snapped? The nursing staff promised to keep an eye on him.

Was this the end of the beginning or the beginning of the end?

Seventh Inning Stretch

It was a beautiful Sunday morning; my husband and I headed to a Twins ball game at the new Target Field in Minneapolis. We met our oldest son and his wife, anticipating a fun family outing.

In the second inning. my youngest sister called. When she came to check on Dad, she found him agitated and not talking. They headed to the hospital.

Should we leave the game early? I wavered between annoyance and guilt. It seemed like only yesterday I had rushed to the emergency room for one of my mother's incidences. Was this hospital run starting over again?

Because we had taken the light rail to the game, our son and his wife drove us home shortly after the seventh inning stretch. I headed to the hospital for what was one of the worst nights of my life with Lewy. One of my worst nights so far.

By the time I met my sister there, he was lying in a gurney in the ER, wearing only a hospital gown and a thin sheet. He was literally incoherent, restless, and aggressive. His eyes were wild, not focusing. The nurse told me not to let him grab my hand—they were afraid of his grip.

I didn't care. I held his hand. I knew he was still strong from all those years of physical labor. But I wasn't afraid; I knew he wouldn't hurt me.

The evening wore on. Tucked between two curtains in the emergency room, my sister and I took turns sitting by him, calling the other two sisters, and huddling in a corner wondering what would happen.

He just wouldn't calm down. What was going on in his head?

Finally, the medical staff suggested giving him an antipsychotic med, then they would move him to a room. We called Sister 2, the therapist, for advice. She said to tell them no anti-psych meds. Research indicates anti-psych meds, usually used in healthy adults with mental illness, causes more confusion in patients with dementia.

We told the medical staff no; we did not consent.

Time wore on. What to do?

The nurses said it was necessary—how else would they deal with extremely agitated patients?

Sister 4 and I huddled in the corner—what to do?

Despite our concerns, we finally conceded, and he was given the meds. It almost immediately calmed him down. Around midnight they checked him into a hospital room, and he slept soundly.

We went home to bed to wonder, What next?

After keeping Dad overnight in the hospital, they sent him home the next day with more medications and instructions for the assisted living staff.

Within two days I received a call at work from the head nurse at the Plaza. When the aide came in to give him his morning meds, she found him lying next to the bed glassy-eyed, the shower running.

The nurse had called 911, the ambulance was on the way, and could I meet him in the emergency room?

"Yes, of course I'll just leave work—again—and head to the hospital."

Did he have a stroke? Or a series of strokes? We never received an answer to that question.

This time the hospital kept him for several days. I am thankful my employer was understanding and flexible. And thank goodness Sister 2 could once again fly home to help manage the hospital situation. They told us to start looking around for a nursing home.

(In what spare time would we hunt for a nursing home? I wondered.)

On Friday, I attended my company's annual Council Meeting in downtown Minneapolis (a major event, where several thousand attendees came from around the world). I had to leave the main gathering to answer hospital phone calls several times. Two items of significance happened that day:

- My company was selling a new jewelry line to benefit our foundation. It was lovely, but I am not prone to impulse spending. However, I was in a fog and impulsively charged $400 worth of jewelry for myself. A friend of mine, whose husband had died at an early age, said she shopped her way through grief. This was my shopping through grief.
- Sister 2 was at the hospital with Dad when they suddenly decided to move him out before the weekend. Had we found a nursing home yet? Sister 2, not familiar with the area, asked if I had any ideas. "Where should they move him?"

No, I had no ideas, no ideas on a nursing home, no time to look, no ideas what to do about my father. It was all moving too fast. I was angry at "the system" (whatever that was), angry that my strong, competent father was reduced to a person with blank, staring eyes, angry I was out of control.

Which is exactly why they have hospital social workers. Late that afternoon Sister 2 called; they had found a place for him. I gave up on attending the Council meeting and drove back to the hospital with my shiny new necklace.

Nursing Home #1

Yes, they had found a nursing home about twenty miles from the hospital. Would we please move him out by dinner time? He was discharged, and Sister 2 and I put him in the car (which was a challenge) and drove him to his new home, where he would be for the next six weeks. He was completely baffled as to what was happening.

For him, it was his temporary new home. For me, it was the house of tears.

I learned to not move a loved one into a nursing home on a Friday evening if it is avoidable.

First, you will encounter the weekend staff. I'm sure the weekend nursing staff were excellent, but generally there are no administrators, physical therapists or social workers on duty. We had to wait until Monday to get Dad evaluated.

Second, they wouldn't let Dad get up and walk until physical therapy visited him on Monday. They had to help him in and out of bed and put him in a wheelchair all weekend.

There were buzzers on the wheelchair and bed, in case he tried to get up on his own. It was his own invisible brick wall.

Not being able to walk on his own made Dad frustrated and angry. (And who could blame him!) It was a bad weekend. We spent as much time as we could with him, wheeling him about, trying to talk to him, watching him shakily eat. The family was broken hearted and frightened.

Finally, on Monday physical therapy assessed him and let him get up and walk. Or should I say he got up and shuffled.

He shuffled back and forth, back and forth, up and down the halls. Lewy is full of surprises, and changes can come fast and unexpectedly.

I was concerned he might walk right out the glass windows.

He barely talked, and when he did it was in a whisper.

But do you know what he *could* do? He could hum hymns and even sing a line or two in a low voice. They say music stays deep in the brain, even through the fog of dementia.

In the beginning, once he got over the shock of moving, Dad was still his charming self to the staff and residents—they loved him! He'd help others when he was able.

Even though my dad could barely speak, he shared his heart with others in his community. I love this poem he wrote years before he was in a nursing home.

I saw a sparrow with a broken wing,
Who sat upon a branch to sing.
She said, "Today I cannot fly
Among the clouds that sail on high."

Though with broken wing I must rejoice,
For God has given me a voice.
To lift up some troubled soul,
Who by my song can be made whole.

The Bible says no sparrow shall fall,
But what my Father knows it all.

So though impaired somewhat today
I'll lift my voice to you and say,
I give the gift I have to give,
To share what I have, so you too can live.

Tears

I recall at least two nights leaving Dad at that first nursing home and crying all the way home.

One night I started to cry when I left his room. I wondered why no one looked at me or stopped me as I walked down the long hall and out the front door with tears streaming down my face. I suppose people often cry as they go out the front door of a care home.

At first, we were hopeful he might be able to go back to the Plaza. The Plaza staff implored us, "Let us try to take care of him, this is his home."

But as the weeks wore on, we realized this was it; there was no going back.

Dad still shuffled through the halls, although his shuffling became a slow gate. As time went on, he could barely form words, much less a sentence. His few words either did not make sense, or they were like those of a small child—hot, cold, water.

Yet another night I found myself crying on the freeway, driving home.

I cried for my strong, independent dad, who should be laughing and telling stories with his buddies.

I cried for past years of family life that were now gone. No more stories about his childhood or what it was like to be in business for himself. No more sharing history.

I cried because I couldn't talk through my feelings with my dad. I always imagined telling him I was hurt when he left my mom, or when he nearly put them into poverty by not paying attention to his business. I imagined him apologizing, and he and I having a time of resolution and forgiveness.

A couple of years later, I was lamenting this point to my youngest sister. She pointed out that men in Dad's generation were not exactly touchy-feely. Kind, caring, but not touchy-feely. He probably had no idea I had all these unanswered questions (and in reality, it would have been far too direct of me to verbalize my feelings.)

I know now he loved me, even though he probably did not understand me, as I did not exactly understand him. A good dance does not have to be in perfect harmony.

Chapter 13

Medications

This chapter is in no way medical advice, always seek the help of a professional physician.

At that time there were a couple of medications prescribed for Alzheimer's. Donepezil (Aricept) is used to treat all stages of Alzheimer's and is believed to boost a chemical in the brain. Memantine (Namenda) is approved to treat moderate to severe Alzheimer's disease. Neither is a cure.

While these drugs were not recommended for vascular dementia, they did give him Aricept for a while. Whether or not it helped, we'll never know.

There was evidence stating that statins may help vascular problems; Dad was on a statin drug for several years. Towards the end of his life, a physician told me the current research showed statins *do not* help prevent dementia or the mini strokes happening in his brain.

A good physician will be schooled in the most current clinical expertise and is more reliable than the internet. However, the sad news is, there are very few other drugs that have been developed to treat dementia.

Antipsychotic Medications

I told you about the first night in the hospital when he was given the antipsychotic medication. The other time he received this medication was in the first nursing home.

I was headed out of town to a work conference. Our normally mild-mannered dad was becoming more and more agitated and resistant. There was one nurse I'll call Pauline who was a no-nonsense kind of person. She knew they were supposed to call me first when they were changing meds, but I was on an airplane and out of touch for several hours. She also could not reach my youngest sister, the alternative person named in the healthcare directive.

So instead she reached another family member who hesitantly gave consent. (I might have agreed to give the medication also, but it annoyed me that they couldn't wait an hour or two to talk to me first.) I later addressed the issue with the head of nursing. They talked to Pauline. They reported back to me because the weekend was coming, they had to get him calmed down for the weekend staff.

Yes, the meds did calm him down, but the sad part was that he became more rigid and withdrawn. And it took many months to get him off the anti-psych medication; he stayed on it the entire time he was in the first nursing home (about six weeks).

You quickly lose control when a family member enters the care system.

The medical team at this nursing home was comprised of kind and caring individuals, but I imagine taking care of sick, declining patients' day after day takes a toll. And the most common way to handle agitation in an institution is to medicate.

Do you ever wonder why you see so many blank faces when you walk into a nursing home? Yes, much of that is due to dementia. But it is also due to antipsychotic drugs, given to calm down the residents. It is called chemical restraint, because restraint via bands or cords is illegal. (It is even illegal to use a bed rail for a nursing home patient.)

It is stressful for all involved.

Reconsidering Medications

I learned more about the elderly and drugs at a dementia conference I attended during my dad's illness. A geriatric physician gave an example of an elderly man (well over eighty) on virtually no medications. The man was hospitalized for heart issues and came home on blood pressure pills, diabetes medications, thyroid pills, blood thinners, and more.

The physician asked why? Why give an elderly person all those meds? What if he didn't receive the blood pressure pills or blood thinners and died of a heart attack?

What if? Are we meant to live on and on, with super-medications or artificial machines?

Was this physician advocating withholding treatment from a person because he or she is older? "Let them die, don't waste money on pills." Of course not! Many medications improve the quality of life for people of all ages. I personally take several prescriptions to improve my quality of life. (Better living through chemistry, we like to say.) This is a deeper, more philosophical question.

When my father was nearing the end of his life, upon careful consultation with his medical practitioners, we gradually pulled him off nearly all his medications, including blood pressure pills, thyroid meds, and more. At the end of his life we agreed we would *only* give antibiotics for infections such as an eye or bladder infection.

I understand if you think this sounds heartless; there was a time I would have thought so also. Believe me, if he died from not having a blood pressure pill, it would have been a blessing.

(You will read later about the end of his life and the mental turmoil surrounding end-of-life issues.)

The burden of being a caregiver is a difficult one to carry. Having to make decisions about medications is tough, even with advice from caring practitioners. At times I felt useless, guilty, frustrated, and helpless.

Once again, do not ever take a loved one off a medication without medical advice. Every situation is different.

More to come later regarding medications—to use, to not use, to discontinue. Tough decisions for the medical team and caregivers.

Chapter 14

Another Move

Dad was just getting settled in the first care home when they let us know he would have to move. He was going downhill mentally, could not talk much anymore, but still wanted to walk up and down, up and down the halls. They were not situated to handle people needing advanced memory care, plus they were remodeling and did not have enough space.

Shortly before he moved, Dad spoke his final complete sentence to his daughters.

Did he say, "I love you"? Or "I don't want to be here"? Or even "Stay with me."?

No, none of the above.

My youngest sister called me over. I put my ear by his mouth. "What's wrong, Dad?" I asked him.

He mumbled something about inappropriate actions he witnessed by the staff.

"What, Dad? When does this happen?" my sister asked.

"Every day, all day. Everywhere."

Most likely not true. People with dementia can lose all their inhibitions. Or maybe this was a Lewy body hallucination?

Where would we find a place for Dad?

Sister 4 and I were hoping to move him to the northern suburbs of Minneapolis, closer to where we lived. But there were only a couple of facilities taking memory care patients, all with long waiting lists.

(One place called me a year after he died to say they still did not have room, but he was still on their waiting list. I said, "Thank you, but you can take him off, he doesn't need nursing care any longer.")

Another complication was the need to find a place that would take medical assistance, should he run out of money. Many places don't take public financing, or if they do, they have a limited number of spaces for those patients. There would be no guarantee he could stay if he did run out of money, and the government had to pay.

A social worker at the first nursing home suggested we check out "AJ's" in Minneapolis. We took a tour of their memory care unit and were immediately impressed. They have halls with various themes for the residents. A central space serves as the nurses' center, the dining area, and the meeting/gathering place where activities can be held. A family-friendly atmosphere prevailed.

After six weeks in the first home, we moved Dad to "AJ's." I'm certain moving again was even more disorienting to him. AJs was centrally located to the three sisters, although not particularly close to any of us. However, under the circumstances it was certainly the best option, and I knew they would work with me on medical assistance when the time came.

Life at AJ's was to become the new normal, and I thought this was okay. We were on a steady state—it couldn't get any worse, right?

Was I ever wrong!

I was also going downhill. I describe depression as "being sucked into a black hole."

Stupid cancer. I was still grieving my mother's death.

Stupid dementia. Watching someone suffer with dementia is like having the hairs plucked out of your head one by one.

Tears and more tears.

Between my mother dying and Dad's decline, and likely from being early post-menopausal due to surgery, I became more and more depressed. I was not a particularly emotional person in the past, but now I cried at the drop of a hat.

Grief rips at your soul. When someone dies, we grieve, sometimes for years. When someone is slowing slipping away from you mentally and physically, the grief is drawn out slowly, repetitively.

I lay in bed several nights, sobbing away. My poor husband did not know what to do other than hold me when I was sobbing.

A sad movie or TV show and my makeup streaked down my cheeks.

Those sappy commercials about homeless dogs—sad, sad, sad.

When I had been depressed previously, I took St. John's Wort, which was just enough to keep me on an even keel. But not anymore.

One day at work my computer wouldn't boot up. My eyes teared up. A co-worker walked in and said, "Are you okay?"

I said yes, but I knew this was not normal. I was not okay.

(Looking back, it is ironic that technology would be the last straw.)

Finally, I went to the doctor and told her what was going on. They called it "situational depression" and prescribed antidepressants.

Why had I waited so long?

Packing Up Again

We let the Plaza know we would be terminating Dad's apartment lease. We had to pack up his remaining earthly possessions, other than the few clothes and items he could have in the nursing home.

I joined my sisters on a crisp autumn Saturday to pack. One very odd situation we found was quite a few end rolls of toilet paper. I wondered why he would hide them in the back of the cabinet. I later remembered a time he ran out of toilet paper, and I had to run to the store to get him a package. This was his way of making sure he never ran out!

By the middle of Saturday, I had a pounding headache. I am not prone to migraines, but I was nauseous and feeling sick. Stress.

My sisters had to take a break and run an errand, so I decided to visit a local craft show. There was a man there giving massages as a fundraiser, $1 a minute. I forked over $20 and had the best head and neck massage ever. It nearly took away my headache. A little self-care will go a long way.

New Home, New Staff

It wasn't just Dad getting used to his new home. In the fourteen months Dad was at AJ's the family spent a lot of time in the facility. It was very nice, there was a library, various rooms we could sit in, they had concerts in the evening and activities during the day. However, not everything was perfect. I had to remind myself that care homes are institutions, made up of people just like you and me. These workers are dedicated to their jobs—people loving to serve and care for seniors. (They are certainly more sensitive and kinder than I am—a wimp who cannot stand the sight of blood, melts in a medical emergency, and would cringe at cleaning up someone's bodily fluids.)

For more ideas on assessing nursing homes or working with the staff, see Part II of this book.

Visiting Dad

Senior care homes often try to provide sensory experiences for their residents. They will give women baby dolls to "mother." Boards are provided with locks and latches for people to fiddle with, along with safe tools or materials. These items offer a sensory experience. Books with colorful pictures are on hand.

My father always liked to read, so I thought I would buy him books about machinery and vehicles for Christmas. Unfortunately, he clearly saw through me; he took one look at those books and threw them—apparently, they were too childlike. Oops. Bad on my part to underestimate my dad. This situation still haunts me.

I later bought him a large book on animal migrations, which I loved and thought he might enjoy. He only stared blankly at the book when we'd go through the pages.

Visiting with Dad could be a challenge since he could barely communicate. There was a nice patio area at AJ's with swings and flowers. I wheeled him out there one sunny day. He whispered a word; I listened closely.

What, Dad?

"Hat"

I forgot to put on his outside hat. I had to run find it for him.

The best times were when another family member came along on visits. When I found my sisters, or other family members at the nursing home, or my husband and I would go together, there would be someone else to converse with, while Dad listened. Especially sweet were the times one of my sons, Lee and Corey, would come along to see Grandpa. Time passed more quickly on those days.

At first when I visited, I'd order a dinner to have with him (yes, their food was pretty good.) I'd eat while he ate, and when he couldn't feed himself, I'd feed him. Eventually that became too difficult, as feeding him required full-time attention. The staff would divide residents among tables of the people who were still lucid and could feed themselves, the residents that needed a lot of help, and the residents that needed to be fed. This way they could facilitate feeding two or three high-need people at the same time. A true art!

When it was just me visiting, I'd read from the Bible, wheel him around to look at the displays, or play music. Hymns played on a recorder seemed to calm him, and we would often leave them on to play in his room when we left. Dad seemed to have no interest in watching TV. As time went on, he would usually just stare straight ahead with what I call "Lewy eyes." (Lewy eyes are a blank stare into nothingness.)

Fourteen months at AJ's are a blur of visits, holidays in the common room, care conferences, and watching him lapse into more silence, more muscle rigidity, and even more blank stares. Shortly after arriving, he had lost the ability to walk, and he eventually lost the ability to even feed himself.

More tears, more mourning, more grief.

Nursing Home Staff

Most of the nursing staff were caring, loving and dedicated. I remember one nurse, a gentleman from the West Indies. He hovered around each of the residents under his care. My sister described him as a bird flitting from patient to patient, keeping an eye on each one.

Another of the day nurses was so kind and caring; she said she cried every time one of her patients died. I believe her; she was so invested in their care.

The head nurse on the floor and I were in frequent contact. She walked me through procedures and any difficulties with my dad, such as accidental injuries to his fragile skin or difficulty in moving him.

We talked about the shortage of nursing assistants and the lack of budget for training. She urged me to tell the world their story and to appeal for more funding and resources for seniors.

There was one frustrating event: both pairs of Dad's eyeglasses were lost right after he moved in. I spoke with the administration staff several times. Eventually they helped pay for a new pair, which we marked with his name right away.

(This inspired me to get Lasik eye surgery, as I had very poor eyesight and feared being blind as a bat in a nursing home someday.)

All in all, we liked and appreciated most of the staff in the second nursing home.

Certified Nursing Assistants (CNAs or "aides") take training for four to twelve weeks (it may vary in different states or countries.) They are low-paid, and many CNAs in this part of the U.S. are from other countries. English may not be their first language. (That being said, I totally admire anyone who moves to another country and has some mastery of a new language—I have never lived more than about forty miles from where I grew up.)

Nearly all the aides, regardless of background, served the residents with loving care. This story isn't about an aide because she was from another country; this story is about an aide and me, and how God works.

There was one nursing assistant I didn't care for; I'll call her Ada. She was clearly unhappy, and at times harsh. (Before you judge me too harshly, remember that having a loved one in a nursing home is like having a child in daycare. You are not there every moment; perhaps you feel protective and/or guilty leaving a loved one in a home. It is your job to defend and guard the care of your loved one.)

One day Dad indicated he had to go to the bathroom before mealtime. Ada was clearly frustrated as she had a schedule to keep. Plus, they did not like taking Dad to the bathroom because he was slow and obstinate and still had a super-strong hand grip.

For this reason, there were supposed to be two aides with him in the restroom.

(In retrospect, he was likely wearing "adult diapers," so it may not have mattered so much if he wasn't brought to the bathroom right at that moment. I did not even think of that being the case.)

Ada wheeled him into his bathroom, and I waited in the hall. Ada looked very cross. She stood outside the door and hollered, "Someone help me—Lee has to go to the bathroom." I was horrified. Another aide came to assist.

I later complained to the head nurse, who had already heard of the incident. She coached Ada to not yell in the hallway. I was protective of my dad and didn't like Ada.

Fast-forward four months. I had not seen Ada around for a while. She reappeared at work one afternoon and took my sister and me aside.

Ada said, "I went home to Kenya to take care of my dad before he died. Now I understand what it is like to have a sick parent." Ada had tears in her eyes, and so did we. This was a lesson in understanding and compassion for all of us.

Why wasn't I more gracious to Ada? I could have said, "Ada, I know you work hard, and I appreciate all you do to take care of my dad. I imagine it's hard for staff to understand how difficult it is for people like me to see their loved one deteriorate."

A medical care team from one of the local hospitals was assigned to Dad. The doctor came monthly, and the nurse practitioner came more frequently.

Monthly care conferences were held with the staff and the nurse practitioner. At one care conference, the practitioner had an announcement: *"We have determined your dad has Lewy body dementia."*

Lewy body dementia. I remembered that it was the disease they thought my friend Karen's husband suffered from before they diagnosed him with frontal lobe dementia.

Lewy and Dad were becoming one at that point. Was I talking to Dad or talking to Lewy?

I remember feeling more confused . . . and number. I still didn't know much about Lewy body dementia. But I witnessed the impact of Lewy growing in his brain.

It seems (from my viewpoint) that Lewy body dementia represents the worst of Alzheimer's and the worst of Parkinson's combined. It is the loss of memory and brain function like Alzheimer's, combined with the rigidity and stiffness of Parkinson's disease.

It was worse than my mother's cancer—once her kidney cancer returned with a vengeance, she died within three weeks.

Lewy body dementia affects almost every system in the body—cognition, sleep, physical, and behavioral. It may cause hallucinations or Parkinson's-like rigidity and can affect bowel and bladder control, blood pressure, and temperature regulation.

Each disease takes its own course, and I am not saying my loved one's horror is any worse than anyone else's. Pain and suffering are just brutal. I watched the horror of Lewy overtake my dad's body and brain.

As time went on, Dad couldn't even lift a piece of bread to his mouth. He was carried in and out of bed with a hydraulic lifter. While this is a great invention for staff, I just could not watch. I'd wait to say goodnight until he was safely tucked into bed. Dad would be turned over periodically.

Uncle Sam Gives

In September 2011, Dad ran out of money. Of course, I knew this was coming, so I was prepared. (Thanks to my mother and her bookkeeping, I still had the records from when I initially applied for Medical Assistance years ago.) Finally he was approved, and the government paid his nursing home bills of over $6,000 a month. (I am glad he did not now, he always took great pride in providing for his own, just like the verse he had underlined in his Bible.)

When my parents sold the house in July of 2006, they gave each of us four daughters $1,000. (This was basically our entire "inheritance.") For five years, I wondered what would happen if my parents ended up needing MA, as the government has a five year "look-back" period. Would we have to declare that they "gifted" us this money? I asked my oldest son who works for the county. He said yes, we would have to declare any significant funds they gave away within the last five years.

Note the date he began receiving Medical Assistance—September 2011. The five-year period ended July 2011.

Coincidence? Luck? No, I don't think so. I believe God was protecting my parents, just as he had promised, and he was also looking out for us sisters, as this $1,000 was basically our entire "inheritance".

Why Dad? Why Me?

At least I wasn't crying too much anymore. I suppose the anti-depressants were working. Maybe I was cried out. I could just pray and try to survive.

Managing my father's care for the fourteen months at AJ's was like trying to manage the care of a child, only worse. Children are striving for independence and achieve it little by little. My father was striving for independence and was losing it by leaps and bounds.

A part of me tried to spend as much time with him as possible. I'd go to visit him at least one night after work and on the weekend. But part of me was angry and resentful. Taking care of my mother had been different—not always easy, but more emotionally doable.

My dad was becoming someone I did not know. Eventually he was dressed, bathed, fed, and diapered by others. He did show some recognition when we visited but could say few words. Mostly his eyes were blank and hollow.

Dad used to have the most vibrant blue eyes. Now they were just hollow and gray.

I prayed for mercy; I felt as though whatever I did wasn't good enough. I needed to know that God understood, and what I did was good enough. How could I keep the mental fortitude to witness this horrible transformation and keep going when I didn't feel like I could?

In the Christian Bible and Jewish Torah, the fourth of the Ten Commandments reads: "*Honor your father and your mother, so that you may live long in the land the Lord your God is giving you*" (Exodus 20:12).

The Muslim Quran reads: "*Be kind to your parents if one or both of them attain old age in thy life, say not a word of contempt nor repel them but address them in terms of honor*" (17:23).

Hindus teach: "*The father, mother, teacher, elder brother and one's provider - these five are considered as one's superiors. He who desires prosperity should revere these superiors at all times by all means, even if he loses his life. The son should be devoted to them and make their care his first priority.*"

Many other religions and world views teach the value of honoring one's parents.

I knew in my head this was right, but my heart was still cold at times.

Then I read the following written by Paul to Timothy: "*But if a widow has children or grandchildren, these [the children or grandchildren] should learn first of all to put their religion into practice by caring for their own family and so repaying their parents and grandparents, for this is pleasing to God . . .Give the people these instructions, so that no one may be open to blame. Anyone who does not provide for their relatives, and especially for their own household, has denied the faith and is worse than an unbeliever*" 1 Timothy 5:4, 7-8.

I came to understand that I took care of my dad because I loved him, but also because God called me to do so. When God calls us, and we listen, He will give us strength and mercy. Whatever your faith (and I hope you have a faith), listen to the wise teachings about caring for your elders.

These passages do not say we take care of our parents or grandparents when it is easy, or when they are pleasant to be around. It doesn't say if our parents were mean and abusive in their previous years, we are off the hook.

I often moved between guilt, resentment, anger, and sorrow. Lewy wreaked havoc with all our lives. My dad couldn't walk anymore. No need to dance around the issues now because Lewy was upon us full bore.

Did You Brush Your Teeth Today?

While I was caretaking for my parents, my dentist of twelve years acquired prostate cancer. He quit his practice and sold it to another dentist. Somehow, I fell off their recall list for my usual six-month checkup.

In my flurry of caretaking, I completely forgot to go to the dentist for a year and a half. Ugh—I was a faithful caretaker of my teeth, going in for six-month visits religiously, until I got lost in the caretaking world.

My dad seemed to have a dental phobia, at least when I started getting involved in his teeth care in 2006. He was missing a lot of teeth and when I started getting involved, we had dental issues galore. I don't know when he had had his last dental visit. The first cleaning and subsequent visits created a lot of grumbling on his part and certainly made me more of a culprit in his misery. Dad was missing quite a few of his molars; the dentist said it was surprising he could even chew.

The Alzheimer's Association website contains excellent tips on how to assist a loved one with oral mouth care. They advise:

> *As Alzheimer's progresses, the person with dementia may forget how to brush his or her teeth or forget why it's important. As a caregiver, you may have to assist or take a more hands-on approach. Proper oral care is necessary to prevent eating difficulties, digestive problems, and infections.*[6]

Fortunately when Dad entered the nursing home, taking (or shall I say dragging him) to the dentist came off my list of responsibilities. A dental service came right into the home and sedated Dad when he was due to have his teeth cleaned.

If you are tempted to put off your own dental care, take this advice from Absolute Dental to heart:

> *Bacteria from the mouth can easily get into the bloodstream and cause infection and inflammation wherever it spreads.*
>
> *Substances that are released from gums inflamed by infection can actually kill brain cells and lead to memory loss. Dementia and possibly even Alzheimer's disease can result from gingivitis when the bacteria in the mouth spreads to the nerve channels or enters the bloodstream.*
>
> *Taking care to prevent oral health problems like gingivitis and periodontal disease can go a long way toward decreasing the risk for more serious health problems throughout the body.*[7]

The article goes on to describe how poor oral health can affect the heart, the brain, respiratory infections, diabetes, and more.

Much as I'd like to blame my Dad's dementia on poor oral health, the evidence isn't conclusive. But then again, like our mothers and dental offices always say: *Brush and floss your teeth!*

Chapter 15

North Winds Coming

The Song of the Wild Goose

Wispy clouds across the sky,
The wild geese are flying high.
I feel the north winds coming down,
They blow the leaves about the ground.

Those mighty honkers calling me,
To come away with them and see;
And know the places that they go,
Where the pleasant breezes blow.
O wild goose, as you fly so high,
And race the winds across the sky,
I feel you pulling me away,

But I cannot leave 'till another day.

Just now I cannot join your flight,
'Cause other shackles hold me tight.
But in my heart with you I'11 be,
'Till I find life's sweet serenity.

Several years before my parents needed all the care, I went to graduate school. One night the topic in my ethics' class was end of life. Our professor showed three different movie clips, and we discussed the various scenarios:

- A young person in a coma, clinging to life via a feeding tube and ventilator: Should the family keep her "life" going just in case she came back one day? What about the cost of the treatment, likely being shared by taxpayers?
- An elderly woman facing the inevitable end: Should she be given feeding tubes, hydration, other medications? Who should decide?
- A young man paralyzed by an accident wanted to die. He had no control over his body. Would it be right to withhold treatment so he would eventually die?

After four hours of discussing the pros and cons of these scenarios, the professor asked if we should continue discussing end of life in the next class. Twenty pairs of eyes looked at him, horrified, and twenty heads shook "no." We had had enough of that depressing subject. He concurred.

I didn't realize this was God's way of preparing me for very hard decisions.

We had the proper paperwork in place to allow us to make end of life decisions for Dad. But end-of-life decisions are not as simple as "Do we pull the plug or keep him/her going?" We progressively had to make decisions such as:

- Do we treat skin injuries? Of course.
- Should we continue his antidepressant? His blood pressure pills? Thyroid meds? We eventually weaned him off most medications.
- Should they give him antibiotics? We decided they should only give him antibiotics for comfort care, such as for eye infections or bladder infections (common in the elderly). We would withhold antibiotics for any sign of pneumonia (also very common, especially when the elderly aspirate).
- Would he be resuscitated with CPR? Intubation? Absolutely not, he was DNR (do not resuscitate).
- Often towards the end of life, dementia patients aspirate their food. If he couldn't eat, do they put in a feeding tube? We decided no. There was an elderly woman in my dad's unit who couldn't talk, couldn't walk, and was clearly near the end of her life. Her family had a feeding tube inserted into her stomach. I wondered why. Despite the feeding tube, she died before my dad.
- Do we hydrate intravenously? That one was tough. Is hydration comfort care or life-extending? I agonized over this question with the head nurse. She gently explained in his situation hydration would be life-extending. Did we want his life extended? Do we want him to be uncomfortable and thirsty? Ask me later.
- On and on it went.

Stop. Just Stop!

My head was screaming, *"Stop asking me all these questions!"*

My heart was aching. Lewy was growing, taking over our lives. When I wasn't at the nursing home, I was waiting for the next call, the next report, the next set of questions.

Lewy lived in my dad's body, and in my head.

Several years before all of this happened, I was on a trip with a good friend, Lori. Her mother was suffering from Parkinson's disease. During our vacation, her brother called several times. Lori's mom was in the hospital, going downhill. Lori debated on flying home, but we ultimately finished our trip.

"I pray my mom will die," she revealed.

Secretly, I was horrified—who would pray their parent would die? Are not life and death in the hands of God?

A portion of Job 1:21 is often quoted in this context: "*He said, . . . the Lord gave, and the Lord hath taken away; blessed be the name of the Lord.*"

I was naïve. While this Bible verse is is true, I do not think God meant for people to live forever on artificial means with modern medicine extending a painful life.

Fast forward several years. I reminded myself that death for a Christian is merciful since the hope of an eternal home far surpasses the ugliness of this earth.

The apostle Paul wrote in Philippians 1:21, "*For to me, to live is Christ and to die is gain.*" I believe that is true.

And yes, I do believe the Lord gives and the Lord takes away, and absent dramatic methods of extending life, God will take his children home in His perfect timing.

Nevertheless, for much of fourteen months I prayed God would take Dad home to heaven.

Winter in My Heart

Minnesota mid-winter is dark and cold. There was no joy over the holidays in late-2011. Would this miserable winter ever end? Would Lewy, like the cold, heartbreaking Minnesota winter, keep our hearts frozen forever? Was there hope for spring?

In this land of ice and snow,
Where the northern winds do blow,
No flowers on this day I see
Their scented beauty for you and me.

But white is pretty and we have a lot
Covering almost every spot
From the roof up on my house
To the tunnel of my field mouse.

But soon those winds will turn around
And melt the snow from off the ground,
Where flowers and grass will soon abound.
So many birds we'll see and hear,
And lilacs and tulips soon appear.

The family spent Christmas at the nursing home. Was there much left behind those clouded gray eyes?

Christmas is such a special day
With trees and gifts and things;
It fills your being with hope and love
To hear of all these things.
Tinsel and boughs and merriment

Give some their holiday flair,
But my greatest joy of Christmas
Is knowing that you care.
So whatever Christmas means to you,
And whatever things you do,
You've done the greatest thing for me,
By being just plain you.

At least we were there, and Dad—what was left of him—was still with us. A warm, breathing dad.

Here is Dad with his mind and body savaged by Lewy body dementia on that last Christmas.

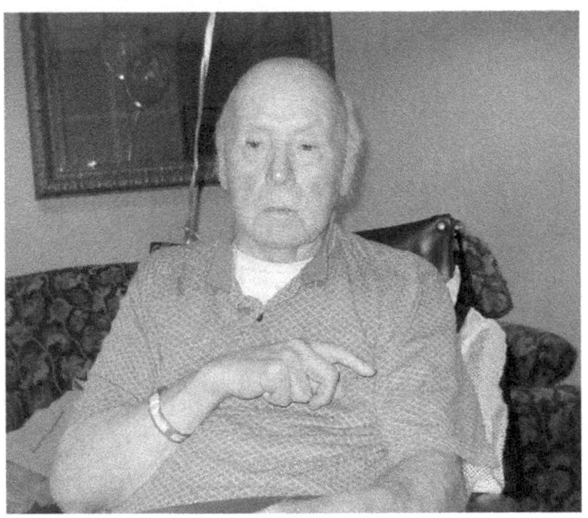

The Last Christmas

About halfway through the afternoon Dad choked on his food, and the nurse came and put him to bed.

We believe he knew us until the end. There was a smidgen of recognition when we kissed him on the cheek. We Skyped with Sister 2, and tears seeped out of his eyes.

In early 2012 he was put on hospice care right there in the nursing home.

Hospice care is awesome. This hospice program was through the local healthcare system treating him. He could get showers several times a week, instead of just weekly. (Of course showers were probably not all that wonderful at this point in his life.) Volunteer musicians and chaplains would visit. The only trouble with hospice care is that it ends, either because the person gets better and is taken off hospice, or they pass away.

The phone calls from the nursing home staff came more frequently. During that cold January, family members trekked in and out of the nursing home.

At a care conference in early January the medical team said he could have another month or two to live.

But only God knows when the end will come.

You never know the last time you will see a loved one.

The Coldest Night

One night towards the end of January, I left work at 4:30, my usual time. It was already dark by the time I reached the care home. There were plenty of parking spots Wednesday evening, since no one wanted to be out in the below-zero Minnesota winter.

There was something to look forward to on this visit. A concert was scheduled downstairs; it would give us something to do.

We stayed at the concert a short time. Dad just stared straight ahead, with no reaction. I did find it interesting that he always sat erect in the wheelchair. No slumping over for Dad.

I wheeled him back up to his floor. The usual guilt set in:

How long should I stay?

Would it be okay to leave before it was too late in the evening?

I knew I should stay longer, and I hated to leave him. But my heart was so heavy, I could hardly bear to see him in this state.

My husband, John, ever *my* caregiver, would have a hot dinner waiting for me at home. I could not have made it through those days without my husband taking care of me.

Lewy was growing in Dad's brain at full bore. Maybe Lewy *was* his brain at this point. I said goodbye and left him sitting erect in his chair, staring straight ahead, in the care of the nurse.

Still sad. Still feeling guilty.

Two days later, Friday evening, I received a call from the nurse. "Your father is especially lethargic tonight. He doesn't want to eat. His blood pressure is up. We just wanted to let you know."

"Is this the end?" I asked.

"We don't think so but call back before you go to bed." I alerted my sisters and debated on driving in the dark and cold to the nursing home. I decided to wait until the later call.

I called back at 10:00 p.m. "How is Lee?"

"Better. He rallied and ate a little soup. He is sleeping now."

I sent my sisters a progress report and decided to go the next morning.

It is never good when your phone rings at 2:00 a.m.

"Hello?" I sleepily answered.

"Yes, Ms. Poland, I am sorry to report your Dad did not make it." It was an unfamiliar voice with a slight accent.

Didn't make it? I thought in my fog.

Didn't make it to dinner?

Didn't make it to the bathroom?

"What do you mean?" I asked, in denial.

"I'm sorry, Ms. Poland, your father passed away during the night. The nurse checked on him, he was sleeping, and a half hour later he was gone."

"Oh. Gone."

"What do you want us to do?"

"Umm, I'll call you back."

I was numb. I called my sisters one by one. One sister thought she might drive to the nursing home. Why hadn't we prepared for this moment?

Another round of calls.

We decided to let them take his shell to the morgue.

It is ironic that our father died in his bed. Years ago, Dad told me he had a deal with God—when he died, he would just pass peacefully in his sleep. That is what apparently happened. (I didn't know a person could make such a deal with God!)

We also concluded that he slipped away during the night because he didn't want his daughters gathered around the bed weeping and wailing, like we did when our mother passed. (Okay, we are Scandinavians, not a whole lot of wailing was going on. But there was weeping.)

Yup, that would be our dad, stubborn and independent to the end.

Lewy won the battle, but I know Dad had a big smile and twinkling blue eyes when he ran to Jesus.

When I walk with my Redeemer
By the river pure as light,
I shall sing a song of glory, of joy
And pure delight.
O for the day of blest rejoicing
When our loved ones we will meet,

And we'll walk with precious Jesus
on heaven's golden street.
Come, let's tell it to the lost ones,
So they too will know His love,
And join the happy throng in heaven
With the Father up above.
All together with the Savior,
Safely in the fold
Because a faithful, loving brother with the Word
went and told.

On Calvary's lonely cross He died
Crown of thorns, spear pierced side
Spikes through bleeding feet and hands
Forsaken of God, rejected by man
Buried in a borrowed tomb
Man's salvation surely doomed
But wait, the Father from above
Came with grace and eternal love
He sent an angel to remove the stone
From between the cross and the throne
Jesus came forth in victory
Eternal life for you and me
Soon the waiting will be over
And we'll be with Him forevermore.

Our Final Words

I was the last one to walk up to the coffin before they closed the lid. Seventy pairs of eyes watched me. The perfume of flowers penetrated the air.

We had our "final words," my father and me. I spoke and imagined he agreed. What I did not know was that those final words would forever change me.

Words I wished I could have said to him years ago.

Healing words. The healing that continues now, seven long years later.

I looked at him and said out loud:

"Okay, Dad, this is it. You are not going to be angry with me anymore, and I'm not going to be angry with you."

Yes, those were my final words with Dad. The shell of Dad.

The anger dissolved like an ice cube on a hot day. Did I immediately forgive him for all ills, real or imagined? Had I not forgiven him earlier?

This moment was about forgiveness, but it was about so much more. It was about harboring misunderstanding, frustration, and resentment in my heart. I can barely explain this— I just know that I was able let go and celebrate my Dad's amazing life.

Funerals are for celebrating life on this earth and for saying good-bye. For me, it was an end and a beginning. It was the end of our somewhat rocky, somewhat loving father-daughter dance. I was and would always be his #3 daughter, his little girl.

Dad was in heaven, and all was forgiven on his side. He could not be mad at me for taking over his finances or for selling the house and moving him into places he didn't want to live. And making him go to the dentist!

Lewy was defeated. Dad was whole again.

How could I do any less? I turned from the casket and had a great big sigh of relief. I sat through his funeral without a tear.

Our Generous Dad

There was the generous side of Dad, a side I didn't fully appreciate until his funeral. My parents were never wealthy, and certainly for the last twenty-five years of Dad's life he lived on a limited income, trying one job to the next. But he was a giving man, sharing what he had.

More than one person approached us with stories, such as our close friends "the Vickers." Years ago, Mr. Vicker had a heart attack and couldn't work. Dad walked into their house, handed Mrs. Vicker $200 (in 1970s dollars) to hold the family over. He walked out without saying a word. Mrs. Vicker told this story to our eldest son at my dad's funeral, and during the eulogy, Lee told this story about his Grandpa Lee.

(Lee is my stepson, and I had pointed out to my dad how handy it was that I acquired a grandchild named Lee right off the bat! Dad was thrilled, and my parents embraced Lee just the same as their other grandchildren).

The pastor friend who had performed Mom's funeral told us a comforting story about Dad. Like the Good Samaritan in the Bible, Dad paid attention to "beggars." Every time Dad spotted a person with a "Need Food" or "Help Me" sign on the side of the road, he would pull over. "If your dad had a nickel in his pocket, he would give the needy person his last nickel."

Dad had told me a story about a time he was working in Duluth, Minnesota. He met a woman who couldn't afford to buy groceries for her children. Dad was quite a friendly guy; apparently, he didn't frighten her because she gave him her address. He bought groceries and milk for her kids and dropped them off at her house.

How many more of these stories could be told about Dad? How many people benefited from this kind, generous man? We do not know the whole story on this side of heaven.

His story is all the sadder knowing Lewy stole his mind and body.

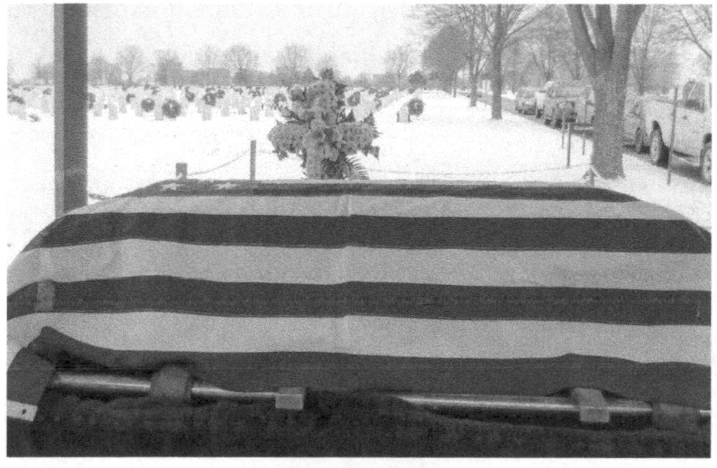

Fort Snelling

Blessings

There is joy in knowing Dad is with his Lord, Jesus Christ. My niece sang the song "Blessings" sang by Laura Story during the funeral. (Another good listen on YouTube.) The song asks if rain, storms, and difficulties are God's mercies in disguise?

What if the storm is a mercy in disguise? What if we did learn to praise God, no matter what?

Dad was buried with full military honors at Fort Snelling National Cemetery.

So much grief, so much pain. Dementia leaves a path of regrets and heartache in its wake.

The week after Dad's funeral I went to California for a conference. My husband flew out at the end of the week, and we spent a long weekend in San Francisco. I was just numb.

Uncle Sam Takes Away

I had to process Dad's outstanding bills and complete the paperwork for his "estate." I could not find any specific information on what could be included in final funeral expenses versus. what the state needed back, so I had asked friends to make food for his funeral lunch.

We ended up having to pay $1,600 back in settlement of his "estate." This is because for the last four months of his life, Medical Assistance covered his nursing home expenses. Had I known then what I know now, I could have used the $1,600 for his funeral lunch as part of his final expenses.

I always knew I wanted to write a book about my dad, me, and Lewy. It took me nearly seven years to write a blog about the experiences. I then decided to turn my blog into this book, in hopes I can help others through the pain of dementia.

Retrospect

Looking back, I understand that my parents were just people on this journey of life, trying to do their best. Back when they were young, there was little talk therapy, support groups, or even antidepressants. Men of Dad's generation were World War II veterans, survivors of horror and creators of a new world order.

My father did not go around speaking his heart; he lived out his beliefs. Sometimes he stumbled, sometimes he sinned—we all do.

There is no righteous or perfect person on this broken earth. We are only made right through Jesus.

Despite Dad's talk about "women-libbers" (which got more pronounced as Lewy took over), he was way ahead of his time in promoting women in many ways. He was proud of his daughters and their accomplishments in both work and at home.

He helped rescue at least one woman from an abusive husband. He gave a woman with cancer my bicycle, so she could enjoy her last months with her scarf blowing in the wind. A woman with a broken background helped keep his side businesses such as glass grinding and sign making straight when he could not. (She helped me find the "lost pot"!)

I am like my dad in many ways—a stoic Norwegian, weathering the storms of life. Somewhat of a workaholic, I am compulsive and committed to whatever I take on. I also strive to be like him in other ways—generous and forgiving.

Throughout his life, whatever the storm, Dad loved God and strove to share the Good News of Jesus Christ.

Part II –

Reflections and Helpful Tips for Caregivers

Reflections

As I look back on my dad's final years of life, I think about "what could had been".

I wish I had been more straightforward with Dad in the early days of his dementia, especially about driving. Many years ago, I read a book about codependency. One concept stood out: Do not make decisions based on other people's anger. Yet I made decisions based on my dad's anger and frustration. We were enmeshed in the father-daughter dance that happens when a strong-willed father raises a daughter who learns to cope by "dancing" around the issues. I didn't want to tackle the inner me; thus I avoided confrontation.

Eventually I learned that this new dad, the dad with dementia, was no longer capable of making rational decisions. The old dad wouldn't drive dangerously, or let the house get run down, or give me his checkbook and then get mad when I helped him manage the money. The new dad, the dad with vascular dementia and Lewy lurking in the background, was still strong-willed, the dad of four daughters, the dad who always thought he knew best. My heart was still reacting to the old dad, even though my head said, "Do something!" I wish I had been kinder and more understanding to the new dad.

If you are a spouse taking care of a loved one with dementia, read Martin J. Schreiber's book, *My Two Elaines: Learning, Coping, and Surviving as an Alzheimer's Caregiver*. This former governor of Wisconsin is an advocate for caregivers and persons with dementia.

I wish I knew then what I know now about how to deal with dementia. I now follow caretakers on Twitter who struggle with a parent with dementia. Through this I found The DAWN Method developed by Judy Cornish. Judy is the founder of the Dementia & Alzheimer's Wellbeing Network (DAWN®) where she shares person-centered care and support for aging in place. Judy teaches how to meet the needs of the dementia patient by understanding their emotional needs.

You will find resources regarding caretaking and dementia on the resources page on my website, www.nancyrpoland.com. I also receive and post recommendations for organizations, websites, or books that will help others.

What did I learn from parental caretaking? I learned about love and forgiveness, and I learned to care for my mom and dad, even when I did not feel loving. I am a practical, pragmatic, and rational person. When events did not fit nicely into the boxes I created, I was left frustrated and confused. Ultimately, love had to win the battles.

Most of all, my faith in God grew by leaps and bounds. I have learned lessons in praising God during the storm. I learned that God is trustworthy—when He promised he would take care of my parents financially; His promises came true. I wish for you a faith in the God greater than you and me.

I learned so much about grace. The ultimate story of grace is the gift of Jesus, who loved us before we knew the meaning of love. My dad would like nothing better than to have you seek the hope found in Jesus.

We face a world of families dealing with dementia. Let us strive for more mercy, grace, and understanding when we come face-to-face with those suffering with Lewy and other dementias. For our friends who are caretakers, let us extend a helping hand. When we are a caretaker, may wc not deny others the chance to reach for our hand.

Helpful Tips for Caregivers

A work colleague just asked me what she should do about her mom, who has dementia, and is going downhill fast. It made me think, what should a caretaker do first? Whether your loved one has dementia, cancer, or any other long-term illness, there are several steps you can take to improve their quality of life, and yours as the caretaker.

ACTION ITEM: Become familiar with your loved one's medical team(s) and health insurance.

When my mother was 59 years old in 1985, she had a mild stroke. My parents did not have health insurance, and she refused to go to the hospital, as they could not afford the bill. She waited until she could see her doctor the next week. This could have been disastrous, fortunately she had a good recovery.

Insurance and healthcare are becoming more accessible in parts of the U.S.; however, premiums and out-of-pocket payments are expensive. Drug costs are exploding. It is critical to understand and help manage a loved one's healthcare if they cannot. This is a priority.

Medicare coverage and supplemental care plans for those 65 and over can be confusing, and the plans change often. Fortunately, there are knowledgeable resources available, from senior call lines, to classes held by insurance companies, to independent brokers. You may find yourself having to get insurance-smart fast, as I did.

Organize medical information

I was overwhelmed by my dad's various medical teams, and the appointments he made. He had a physician, an eye doctor and a dermatologist (but not a dentist…he hated having dental care and went to the University of Minnesota to get his teeth pulled when they got too bad). Dad was able to keep the appointments straight for a while, but eventually I had to work with him on scheduling. Meanwhile Mom had her own set of issues with multiple conditions to manage. I kept files and notes for the various information. Fortunately, electronic records have made healthcare information available with a login to sites such as MyChart; that is, if you have access to your loved one's information.

Each separate clinic has forms to be filled out to access a patient's information. If your loved one can sign those forms, it is helpful. If not, you will have to rely on power of attorney and healthcare directives.

A couple general points:

- If possible, have someone attend medical appointments with your loved one to provide information and take notes.

- Medical records do not transfer themselves, and even if you ask them to be transferred, they may not reach the correct place. You must follow up to make certain the records reach the proper location.
- Even if you have all your proper paperwork in place, surprises await you. Give yourself a little grace if you miss an appointment, if your loved one turns on the charm at the doctor's office and appears to be in perfect condition, or the medical records do not show up. Life happens.

ACTION ITEM: **Obtain a diagnosis.**

It is important to obtain a diagnosis. Do you suspect your loved one has dementia? There are many different types and they are treated differently. It may not be dementia at all; side effects of certain medications, a low thyroid or vitamin B deficiency can all mimic a brain or mood disorder. Urinary tract infections act differently in older people, often causing agitation or confusion. Find a good physician you both trust to get to the bottom of any unusual symptoms.

The same could be said for skin conditions, stomach pains, headaches or other health issues. Unless you are an all-comprehensive physician, you need to consult the experts to see what is happening.

If your loved one is a veteran or the spouse of a veteran, seek out any veteran benefits available. VA clinics and hospitals offer many advantages for those who served our country; vets deserve to utilize these benefits. The local Veteran's Service Organization, county veteran's office, or VA clinic can help you figure out the best way to obtain assistance for your loved one who served.

ACTION ITEM: Create a safe environment for your loved one.

As we age our senses become less acute. Eyesight or hearing may fail, our sense of balance may get worse, and we get more easily distracted. You may see problems in the home a loved one misses.

Does your loved one live alone? Strongly consider obtaining a "call for help" wearable necklace or bracelet. (Cell phones are not always handy or even practical.) Even though Dad was in an apartment in the Plaza with nursing care available, he fell and was on the floor for hours, or even overnight, before anyone found him. We felt terrible; we had a "call for help" necklace for Mom but thought we did not need one for Dad as he lived in a facility with nursing care available.

Often there are simple things you can do to create a safe environment such as:

- Move rugs or use double-sided tape to attach them to the floor.
- Turn the temperature of a hot water heater down, "lock down" the thermostat.
- Install stair railings if needed (inside or out) and bathtub handles.
- Buy nightlights and plug them into the hallway, bathrooms or other rooms your loved one may wander into at night. I found nightlights that automatically came on at dusk especially helpful and placed them strategically around my parent's home.
- Organize closets and move the dishes or pans they use to lower shelves.
- De-clutter the living area to remove tripping hazards.

AARP and the Center for Disease Control (CDC) have safety checklists online. Your local clinic or county may offer assessments to check for falling hazards in the home.

Driving Safety

Ask yourself, "Would I want my children or grandchildren riding in the car with dad, mom, grandma, grandpa, etc.?" If the answer is no, act. Safety for all involved is the priority; be diligent in addressing the situation. The AARP website has helpful information on driving issues. The local VA will perform drivers' assessments, as was the case for Dad, or you could check with a local rehabilitation facility.

Did you know many insurance companies offer discounts for drivers over 55 who take an 8-hour safety course? Again, check the AARP website, or call your community education program.

Guns

I cannot emphasize the importance of removing guns from the home of someone suffering from dementia, or otherwise vulnerable.

In April 2019 the Minneapolis Star Tribune reported, "Prominent Twin Cities businessman Irwin Jacobs shot and killed his wife, Alexandra, before turning the gun on himself in a murder-suicide Wednesday at the couple's Lake Minnetonka home, the Hennepin County medical examiner confirmed Friday…Dennis Mathisen, a longtime family friend, said earlier this week that Alexandra Jacobs 'had been in a wheelchair for the last year or so and had signs of dementia. Irwin was just distraught over her condition.' "[8]

I cannot begin to imagine the pain this double tragedy caused for the family. Caretaking stress is no respecter of persons. Whether we are rich or poor or anywhere in between, there is a breaking point. We must take whatever precautions are available to provide a safety net for our loved ones.

ACTION ITEM: Do not procrastinate on getting your legal house in order!

This may be the most important information you will read in this book. I do not offer legal advice and this information is no replacement for professional guidance.

For your parents, for yourselves, for anyone within your circle of care, you must get the legal paperwork in line. It is important to do so when a loved one can make and understand these decisions; they must be "of a sound mind." I can say now, we just squeaked by on that "sound mind" business with Dad.

You may need a family meeting to determine who will be the estate executor, who will have financial responsibility, and who will make medical decisions. Caregiving may fall to the eldest child or the one closest to home. You may need to help another relative such as an aunt, uncle or grandparent. Without the proper paperwork, you may find yourself in court seeking guardianship of a loved one. It adds unnecessary legwork to an already difficult situation, and you may find your family having to rely on a non-relative or court for decisions.

Some websites have legal documents where you can access forms, information and advice. This may work in a simple situation, however an attorney will know the laws in your state and can analyze your situation. This is especially important if your circumstance is complex; for example, for a large estate, property in different states, divorce or remarriage, or if a disabled child or adult is involved. Engaging a qualified attorney may be the best money you ever spend.

AARP has great resources for members and nonmembers, as does The American Bar Association. You can find these tools on their websites.

Your county, local VA office, or senior citizen advocacy groups may also be available to recommend legal resources.

One more word of advice: You may want to explore a living trust with your attorney. This is a legal document that may protect assets so you can provide for a loved one's care or retain money for a surviving spouse. A living trust may keep property out of probate court, and can be especially helpful for blended families, remarriages or if one spouse is significantly older than the other.

ACTION ITEM: Make sure your loved one has all their important documents in one placc.

Perhaps you are applying for Medical Assistance or VA benefits, and discover you need a marriage or divorce certificate, a birth certificate, or the house title. If you are fortunate, and have a mother like mine, everything is in one place. If you're not so fortunate, you may have to go on a hunt for paperwork.

And while you are at it…get your important paperwork in order!

Some people hire elder care attorneys to complete government paperwork or pay the bills (although you still need to find all the paperwork to give the attorney). Which leads us to the next point.

ACTION ITEM: Seek out resources to help your loved one and you.

I cannot say this strong enough or loud enough—do not isolate yourself as a caretaker. If someone says, "How can I help?", answer with something specific. "Could you bring a small casserole to Dad once a month?" "Could you stay overnight with Mom next weekend so I can go out of town?" "I need someone to do an internet search on nursing homes—can you help?"

Delegate paperwork or bill paying if that is not your strength. Or maybe you're like me and relish organizing paperwork but get squeamish changing pain patches or cutting toenails; it is okay to find others to do those tasks.

Communities, counties or insurance companies may have respite help, services for seniors, or transportation options. The internet can lead you to all sorts of ideas. If you are stressed out and at your coping limit, call your local doctor's office, and keep calling until someone helps you.

If your loved one has dementia of any type, the Alzheimer's Association, alz.org, is there to help. In the U.S. their 24-hour helpline is 800.272.3900, and there are similar organizations in other part of the world. You can find information and support for people with any type of dementia. Community presentations and self-help groups are also available in many areas.

The Lewy Body Dementia Association (LBDA) in Atlanta, Georgia has information, support, and resources at their website, as does The Lewy Body Society in the U.K.

Even though I am several years out from dealing with Dad's Lewy body dementia, I follow a support group on Facebook for those dealing with Lewy, and carefully offer ideas and support. (Just do not believe everything you read on the internet.)

Nearly every major disease or disability has an association with information and support, from cancer, to arthritis, to multiple sclerosis, and many more. Help is only a click or phone call away. Seek out resources, call your county, senior helplines, whatever it takes to create the best situation.

Caretaking is stressful, do not think you can survive without a village to support you.

ACTION ITEM: Visit assisted living facilities or nursing homes before there is a crisis. Often there are waiting lists; you can add their name even if they never move into the facility.

I am grateful we did not promise either of my parents we would "never put you in a nursing home". I do understand why people make those promises as people, especially the older generation, are terrified of institutions. My advice is do not make promises you may not be able to keep. Dad could not walk, could not toilet or feed himself, eventually he could not even transfer himself into bed, he had to be lifted by a hoist. He weighed about 160 pounds when he died; none of us could have cared for him in our homes. Even if a loved one shrinks, not many of us can lift even 80 pounds of dead weight. There are great reasons to keep a loved one home as long as possible, but sometimes 24/7 nursing care is the safest place for someone with a debilitating illness.

What if you already promised your loved one you would always keep them at home", but you have to go back on that promise? Again, give yourself some grace. My "dad after dementia" was not the same dad as before dementia; he would not have wanted any of us to hurt ourselves, physically or otherwise, caring for him. As painful as it was, I felt a great deal of relief knowing he had 24/7 nursing care available.

An ideal situation for many of us would be to live in a community providing progressive care. When we age, moving from an independent-living apartment, to assisted living, to a nursing home in the same complex sounds ideal.

Unfortunately, life is usually not so orderly. Many places do not take Medical Assistance, or only have a certain percentage of openings for those needing government support. Other places are just too expensive, or there may not be such a facility near your home.

But you can prepare ahead of time by researching options. Medicare.gov is a resource for examining nursing homes; you can search under "nursing home compare" both by state and name of the home.

Many states also offer nursing home evaluations. For example, Minnesota has a "report card" on nursing homes on the Department of Human Services website. See if your state has a similar resource.

In the Nursing Home

When your loved one is in a nursing home, find a way to do "due diligence" by monitoring their care.

- Keep an eye on what is going on; visit at odd hours.
- Be on a first name basis with administration and the head nursing staff.
- Remember your loved one may not be able to speak for him or herself; you need to be their advocate. Speak up, ask questions, but do so kindly and with an open mind.
- Make certain the home knows who has power of attorney on financial issues, who can make medical decisions, and who the backup decision maker(s) may be.
- If you are not informed when there are injuries or illnesses, find out why. Be firm— you want to know everything.

If you live far away, and there are no family members nearby, try to find an advocate to visit your loved one and report back to you. Make sure the staff has your contact information, and dial into care conferences.

Most people who work in nursing homes are there because they love people. However, institutions fail, and people fail. No matter where your loved one lives, everything will not be perfect. Practice diligence—and grace.

- A well-placed basket of granola bars in the staff lounge will go far. Treats on a holiday or donuts on an "any" day are appreciated. You may want to slip a gift card to a special staff member.
- My mother-in-law lived in another state, and my husband and I could only visit her once or twice a year. Even though we could not be there, we would ship cheese and crackers or other treats to the staff.
- Be considerate and respectful. Nursing care is hard work, and most homes are understaffed. Most people are doing their best.

ACTION ITEM: If you are going through a difficult time and suffer from depression or anxiety, don't think it will just go away. Talk to your doctor or a professional.

Are you ignoring your health? Missing dental appointments, no time to go to the doctor, pretending to the world you are okay? Not sleeping? Ignoring your own health is an easy place to slip into when you are caretaking. If you are sick physically, mentally, emotionally or spiritually, you can help no one.

Anti-depressants may be needed, even for a short time. Talk therapy is great, as are self-help groups. An occasional massage will do wonders. Please don't suffer unnecessarily.

If your loved one or you are about to hurt anyone, including yourself, do not hesitate to call your emergency number (9-1-1

anywhere in the U.S., or the National Suicide Prevention Helpline: 1-800-273-8255.)

What else can we do?

Legislate: Ask your legislators to support resources or research in the areas you believe need medical or social advancement. It is easy to send an email to your state or federal representatives.

When I was frustrated with the VA system, I sent several emails to my legislators—it just made me feel better, and I would like to think it contributed to added funding to update the VA systems. Our elected representatives are there to serve the people and want to know the needs of their constituency.

Donate: Consider contributing to a fund supporting research, patients or community education. I recommend you check out any charity online at the Charities Review Council website. Most charitable organizations take memorials in honor of loved ones that have passed away.

Educate: Knowledge is power, and the more you know about the challenges you and your loved one face, the better you can face the situation ahead. From books to websites to community education, there are many ways to find answers and solutions. My website, nancyrpoland.com, has a list of resources.

Conclusion

We have reached the end of this book about our battle with Lewy body dementia, and our father-daughter dance. I could continue with caregiving advice for many more pages, but what would I write about in my next book?

My prayer for you and your loved one is from Psalm 4:1, 3 and 8:

Answer me when I call to you, my righteous God.
Give me relief from my distress;
have mercy on me and hear my prayer...
Know that the Lord has set apart his faithful servant for himself.
The Lord hears when I call to Him...
In peace I will lie down and sleep,
for you alone, Lord, make me dwell in safety.

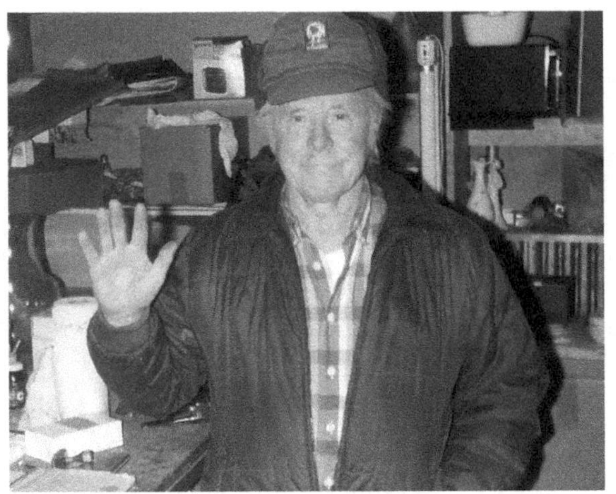

Goodbye Dad, until we meet again

Notes

1 "What is LBD? Who was Lewy?" Lewy Body Dementia Association

2 Williams, Susan Schneider. 2016. "Neurology." *The terrorist inside my husband's brain.* September 26

3 "What Causes Vascular Dementia?" WebMD last reviewed January 23, 2017

4 "Executive Function and Executive Function Disorder." WebMD last reviewed March 25. 2019

5 Huang, Juebin Huang, MD, PhD. 2018. "Lewy Body Dementia and Parkinson Disease Dementia." Merck Manual Consumer Version. March

6 "Dental Care" Alzheimer's Association

7 "10 Health Issues Caused by Poor Oral Health". Absolute Dental, January 26, 2017

8 By John Reinan and Mary Lynn Smith, "Prominent businessman Irwin Jacobs shot wife, then himself, medical examiner confirms", *Star Tribune*, April 12, 2019

For complete references, including websites locations, visit nancyrpoland.com

About the Author

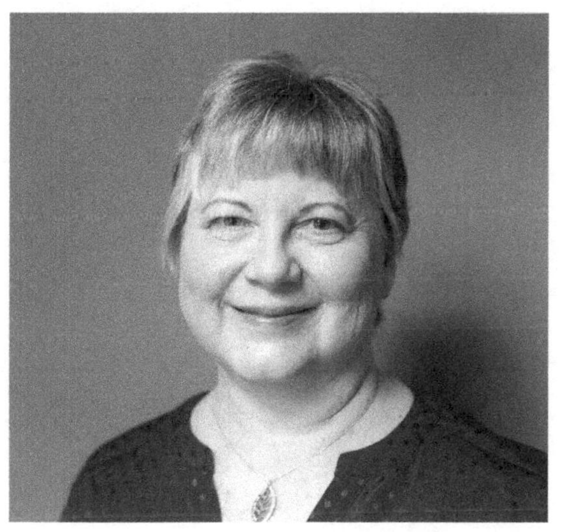

Nancy Poland approaches life with a mix of compassion and practicality. Through her experience as a caregiver for her premature son, a foster child, grandparents and parents, Nancy seeks to better the lives of caregivers and their loved ones through her writing and speaking. A life-long resident of Minneapolis and St. Paul, Minnesota, she and her husband John raised two sons and continue to contribute to their communities. Professionally Nancy manages proposals, contracts and grants; she has utilized her writing and negotiation skills to support both for-profit and non-profit companies. After finishing her master's degree in Health and Human Services Administration, Nancy wrote a thesis on privacy regulations and published an article in the National Contract Management magazine. She also writes stewardship materials, blogs, and communicates via social media through Nancy Poland and Grace's Message.

Printed in the USA
CPSIA information can be obtained
at www.ICGtesting.com
JSHW022333140824
68134JS00019B/1456